28-Day Liver Health Weight Loss Solution

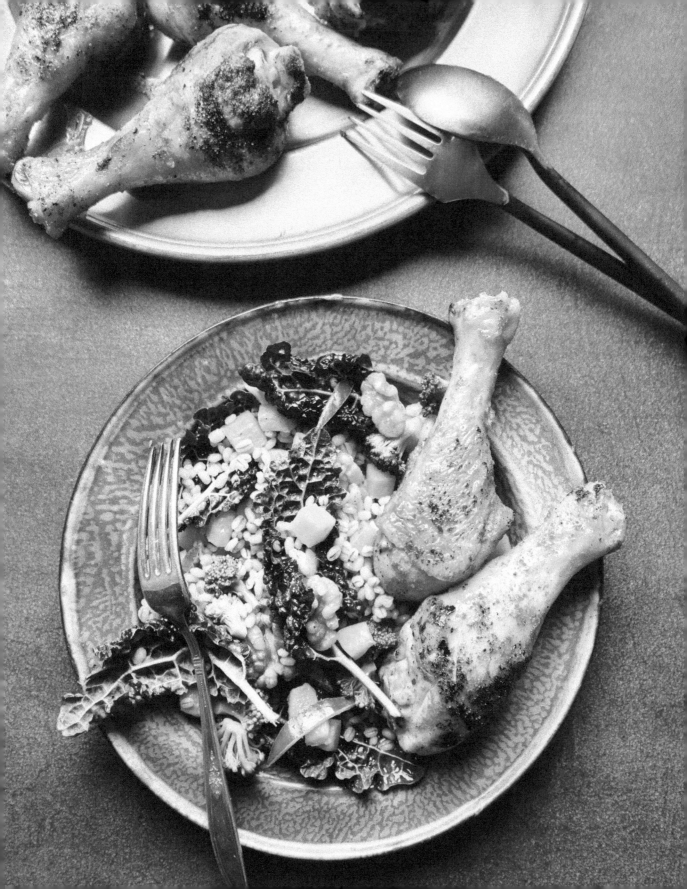

28-DAY
LIVER HEALTH
WEIGHT LOSS
SOLUTION

Fight Fatty Liver Disease with Diet and Exercise

Jinan Banna, PhD, RD

ROCKRIDGE
PRESS

First Rockridge Press trade paperback edition June 2022

Rockridge Press and the Rockridge Press logo are trademarks or registered trademarks of Callisto Media Inc. and/or its affiliates in the United States and other countries and may not be used without written permission.

For general information on our other products and services, please contact our Customer Care Department within the United States at (866) 744-2665, or outside the United States at (510) 253-0500.

Some of the recipes and exercises originally appeared, in different form, in *30-Minute DASH Diet Cookbook, The Diabetic Cookbook and Meal Plan for the Newly Diagnosed, The 30-Minute Low Cholesterol Cookbook, The 28-Day DASH Diet Weight Loss Program,* and *The 28-Day DASH Diet Weight Loss Program.*

Paperback ISBN: 978-1-63878-054-0
eBook ISBN: 978-1-63878-892-8

Manufactured in the United States of America

Interior and Cover Designer: Jill Lee
Art Producer: Hannah Dickerson
Editor: Marjorie DeWitt
Production Editor: Emily Sheehan
Production Manager: David Zapanta

Photography © Thomas J. Story, cover; © Nadine Greeff, back cover (far left) and pp. VI, 2, 16, 26, 42, 122, 134; © Marija Vidal, back cover (center left and right, far right) and pp. II, VIII, 56, 70, 82, 112; © Darren Muir, pp. X-1, 40-41; © Elysa Weitala, pp. 69, 95, 111; © Evi Abeler, p. 96. Illustrations © LeiaSW/Creative Market, p. V; © Charlie Layton, pp. 11, 138-143. Pattern used under license from Shutterstock.com.

012345678910

This book is dedicated to my mother and father, who inspired me to become a health professional and seek to address diet-related chronic conditions.

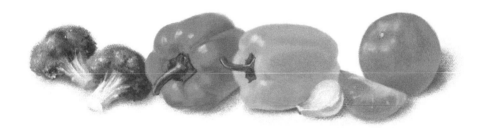

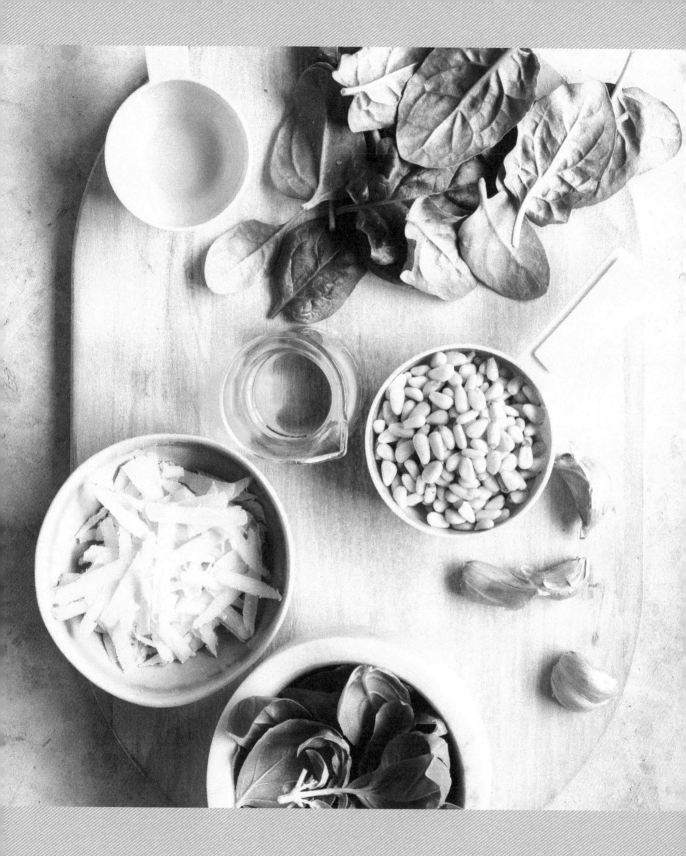

CONTENTS

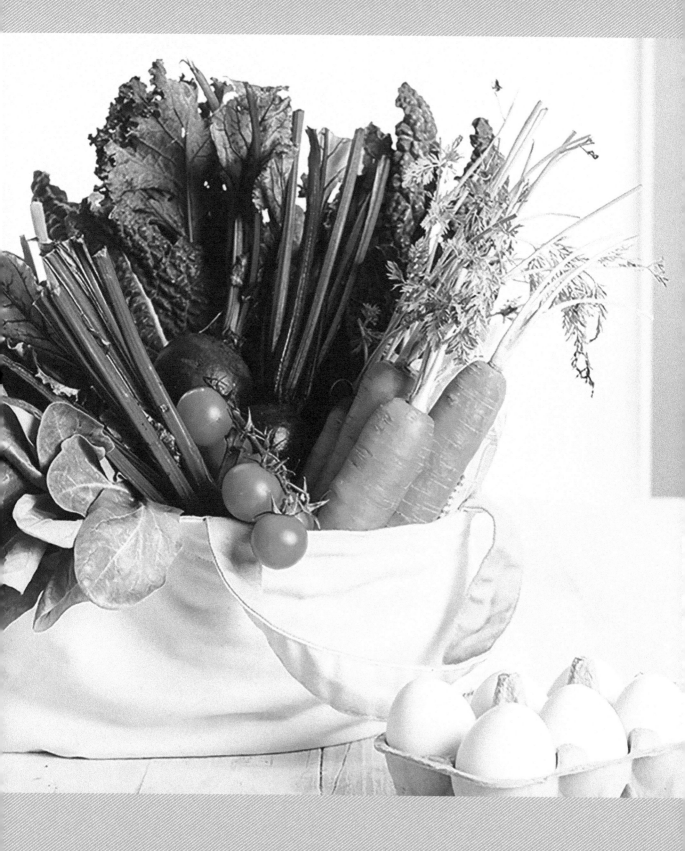

INTRODUCTION

I have written this book to share my professional knowledge as a nutritionist. As a professor of nutrition at the University of Hawaii, and as a registered dietitian with experience helping people improve their diet and lose weight, I am excited to help people understand how diet relates to liver health. Every day in my private practice, I give people easy-to-implement weight loss tips that I am now going to share with you! My clients often come to me confused about what diet to follow to lose weight, so I work with them to help them better understand diet's impact on the body, uncomplicate weight loss, and share the importance of the various nutrients for health. It's a great day when I see clients understand that they don't have to deprive themselves of delicious food to lose weight and become healthier.

Liver health and weight loss can be confusing and challenging, but I'm here to help you get started. This book outlines the basics of liver health and weight loss through a healthy diet. I start by discussing the principles of a liver-friendly diet and how to know what foods to eat. I also talk about comorbidities, like type 2 diabetes and cardiovascular disease, as well as complications of liver disease. I provide meal plans to illustrate how to plan food for each day, and a list of foods to enjoy, avoid, and eat in moderation. The provided recipes will give you plenty of ideas and options for keeping your diet interesting and tasty.

To gain a full understanding of liver health, this book also outlines other topics beyond diet, such as the importance of exercise and sleep, issues with stress, and concerns around environmental toxins. To easily put it into action, I've created weekly meal plans outlining what foods to eat and which exercises to complete. These habits go hand in hand with diet to maintain liver health.

I've provided practical tips for living a healthy lifestyle and plenty of recipes to maintain interest and progress. The key is to develop better food habits through yummy and creative recipes while still allowing yourself the occasional treat. With this book, you will be able to vary your diet, enjoy each meal, and stick to liver health principles. I wish you well on your journey to health.

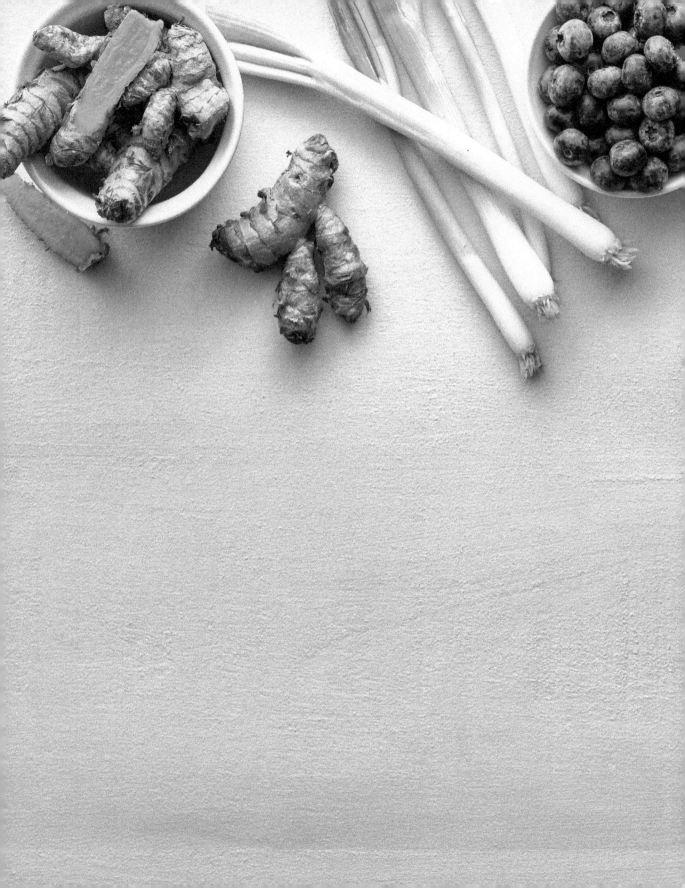

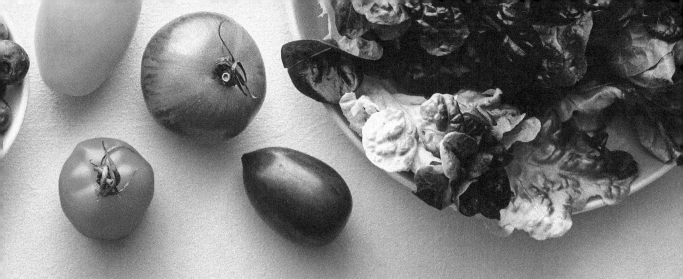

PART ONE

YOUR WEIGHT LOSS PROGRAM

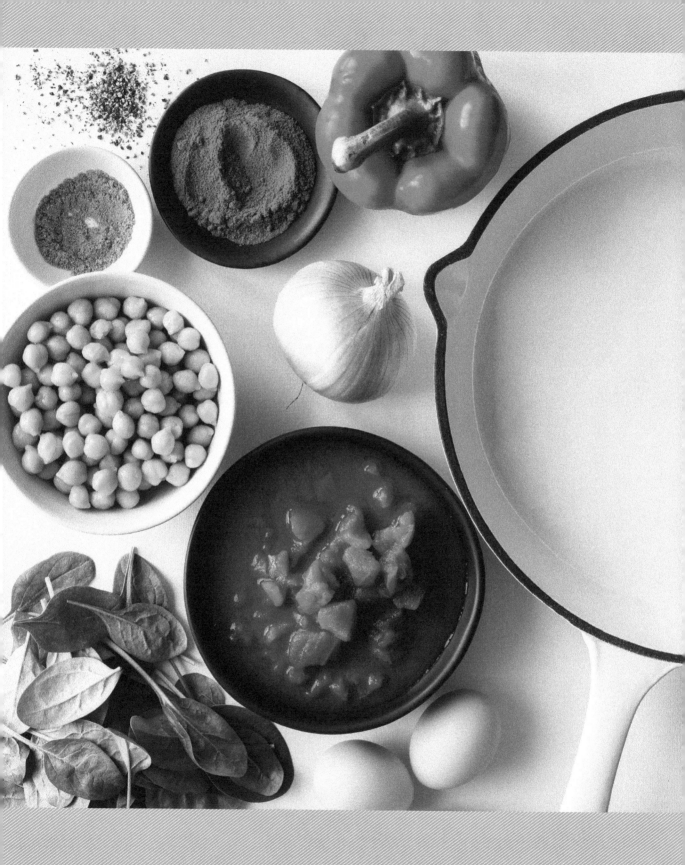

CHAPTER 1

The Healthy Liver Diet

This chapter covers liver disease and the role of weight loss in liver health. It outlines the principles of a liver-friendly diet, including how to balance portions for macro- and micronutrients, and how to determine which foods to eat. Potential comorbidities, such as type 2 diabetes, cardiovascular disease, and sleep apnea, and complications of liver disease are also covered. As with any diet change or weight loss plan, it is always important to consult with a doctor before starting, so please be sure to do so to ensure this plan is right for your individual needs.

A Primer on Liver Disease

This section outlines liver function and the basics of liver disease, both of which are very important concepts to understand before diving into possible treatments.

Liver Function

The liver has numerous roles in the body, including storage of vitamins, digesting food, and processing nutrients. Specifically, the liver aids in the following:

Storage of fat-soluble vitamins. Fat-soluble vitamins are absorbed in the intestine and reach the liver in various forms. The liver stores or metabolizes nutrients such as vitamin A.

Bile production. The liver produces bile, a fluid needed for the digestion and absorption of lipids, which can be thought of as a synonym for "fat." Bile also assists in the excretion of material not excreted by the kidneys.

Maintaining thyroid hormone function. The liver plays a role in thyroid hormone activation, transport, and metabolism.

Drug metabolism. The liver is involved in metabolism or detoxification of substances that are foreign to the body.

Bilirubin metabolism. Bilirubin is a pigment made during the breakdown of red blood cells. This passes through the liver and is excreted. Levels of bilirubin that are higher than normal may indicate liver problems.

Types

There are many different types of liver disease, including hepatitis A, B, and C, auto-immune hepatitis, and cirrhosis. Other types of liver disease are nonalcoholic fatty liver (NAFL) and nonalcoholic steatohepatitis (NASH), both of which fall under the umbrella of nonalcoholic fatty liver disease (NAFLD).

Symptoms and Causes

Liver disease symptoms vary based on the type of disease. For example, hepatitis A. symptoms may include dark urine, fatigue, fever, joint pain, and loss of appetite. NAFLD, in contrast, generally has few to no symptoms.

Causes of liver disease also vary based on type. For example, hepatitis is caused by viruses, and transmission occurs in numerous ways, depending on the virus. Hepatitis A is spread through contact with the stool of an infected person. Hepatitis B is transmitted via contact with the blood, semen, or other body fluids of an infected person. With NAFLD, there are several factors that may increase risk of development, including obesity, metabolic syndrome, high cholesterol, high triglycerides, sleep apnea, and type 2 diabetes.

Complications

One of the main complications resulting from liver disease is cirrhosis, also known as scarring of the liver. Cirrhosis can lead to the following:

- Fluid buildup in the abdomen
- Swelling of the veins in the esophagus
- Confusion and drowsiness
- Liver cancer
- End-stage liver failure

Treatment and Expectations

One of the ways to address liver disease is through lifestyle changes with diet, exercise, and weight loss. Specifically, a calorie-restricted diet and a minimum of 150 minutes of physical activity a week is needed. There are no approved medications to treat NAFLD, so weight loss is the best method to reduce fat in the liver and reduce liver inflammation and fibrosis.

FAQ

Q: How can NAFLD be prevented?

Both a healthy diet and physical activity are key in prevention. A well-balanced diet and reasonable portion sizes is important. Emphasizing whole foods over packaged foods will help keep calorie intake under control. Being regularly active goes along with healthy eating. Both should help maintain a healthy weight, which is a key part of prevention.

Q: Can I drink alcohol if I have NAFLD?

There are a variety of opinions about drinking alcohol if diagnosed with NAFLD. Some research suggests that alcohol should not be consumed because it may cause further damage to the liver and lead to additional fat accumulation. Other research suggests that patients with low fibrosis risk may be able to drink in moderation.

Q: Is NAFLD genetic?

Yes, certain genetic factors increase risk of NAFLD. For example, NAFLD is seen more in Latinx people while being less prevalent with Black people. Looking closely at genetic risk may help diagnose the condition early and develop appropriate treatments.

Q: How common is NAFLD?

NAFLD is a major disease in the United States, and it may be driven by an increase in obesity, diabetes, and insulin resistance. NAFLD affects some groups more than others and is more common in middle-aged or older people than younger people. It can, however, affect children.

Q: Does having NAFLD increase risk of liver cancer?

Yes, NAFLD increases the risk of developing cancer, specifically, hepatocellular carcinoma (HCC). The magnitude of the risk is unclear, but it has been shown that the more severe the disease, the higher the risk of cancer. Cancer risk is highest when cirrhosis, obesity, and alcohol consumption is present. Changes in diet have been shown to decrease risk of liver cancer.

Q: How are NAFLD and metabolic syndrome related?

Metabolic syndrome is a set of risk conditions that occur together and increase the risk of heart disease, stroke, and type 2 diabetes. A metabolic syndrome diagnosis is likely if three or more of these risk factors are present: high blood glucose, low HDL cholesterol, high blood triglycerides, large waist circumference, and high blood pressure.

Q: How does NAFLD affect quality of life?

In the early stages of NAFLD, there may be no symptoms or changes in quality of life. As the disease progresses, however, fatigue or an aching on the right side of the stomach just below the ribs may occur. If cirrhosis develops, symptoms may worsen and include unintended weight loss, yellowing of the skin, or itchy skin, among other possible problems.

Q: What is the difference between NAFLD, NAFL, and NASH?

Nonalcoholic fatty liver disease (NAFLD) is the presence of excess fat in the liver that is not caused by heavy use of alcohol. Nonalcoholic fatty liver (NAFL) and nonalcoholic steatohepatitis (NASH) fall under the umbrella of NAFLD. NAFL refers to the presence of fat in the liver without liver damage. NASH, in contrast, involves liver damage in addition to the buildup of fat. NASH may lead to permanent damage of the liver and liver cancer.

The Role of Weight Loss in Liver Health

Losing weight plays an important role in preventing and reversing liver disease. Those who are overweight are at greater risk of developing nonalcoholic fatty liver disease (NAFLD). It is not completely understood how excess fat promotes changes in the liver, but it is known that weight loss helps reduce risk and fights the disease. Research has demonstrated that even a small weight loss of 3 to 5 percent can lead to fat reduction in the liver. It may also be possible to reduce inflammation in the liver by losing up to 10 percent of one's body weight.

Losing one to two pounds per week is recommended because rapid weight loss may promote inflammation. Even without weight loss, physical activity will likely have a positive effect on the liver. If someone with NAFLD does not exercise, starting to incorporate movement on a regular basis may be a good place to start. Since there are currently no approved medications to treat NAFLD, lifestyle change is the only option for treatment and thus is very important.

The weight loss plan included in this book was created based on the scientific evidence related to diet and liver health.

Five Principles of a Liver-Friendly Diet

There are five recommended steps to a healthy liver. This section outlines those steps and provides ways for easy implementation. Later in this book, we will cover the nitty-gritty of what foods to eat and why.

1. Limit Inflammatory Foods

NAFLD has been connected with low-grade systemic inflammation, so a focus on anti-inflammatory foods is important in preventing and managing the disease. Foods that may contribute to inflammation, such as red meat, should be limited in the diet. A diet rich in plants, vegetables, fruits, beans, nuts, whole grains, olive oil, and fish, known as a Mediterranean diet, is highly recommended because of its positive impact on the liver. Other foods that may cause inflammation are refined carbohydrates, fried foods, and foods high in added sugars. The recipes in this book incorporate anti-inflammatory foods to assist in liver health.

2. Load Up on Liver-Friendly Foods

With liver health, quite a bit of focus is placed on the Mediterranean diet because of its benefits to the liver and its ability to decrease mortality and morbidity. Other foods emphasized in the Mediterranean diet are unrefined cereals, grain products, and nuts. The recipes later in this book are packed with these healthy food items to make this journey as simple as possible.

3. Tailor Nutrition to Your Individual Needs

It is important to be aware of nutritional needs based on individual characteristics like gender, age, height, weight, physical activity level, and existing health conditions. If weight loss is recommended, either to prevent NAFLD or to manage it, monitoring caloric intake is important. How much to eat of any one item will differ based on individual dietary needs, so it is important to consult with a registered dietitian and medical doctor before making changes. For example, if the concern is cirrhosis of the liver, it may be necessary to consume a diet high in calories and protein to prevent muscle loss. A dietitian and doctor can help develop the right diet plan that meets individual needs.

4. Balance Your Meals

A balanced meal with proper portion sizes and a variety of different food groups is important because it helps ensure that there are enough essential nutrients. A plate half full of fruits and vegetables is a great start to proper nutrition. Most Americans don't consume enough fruits and vegetables, which are an important source of vitamins and minerals as well as fiber.

A helpful resource to use in creating a well-balanced meal is the website MyPlate.gov. This website offers an individual assessment tool with personalized resources that will help in the liver health journey.

5. Focus on Fiber

Fiber, a type of carbohydrate, is an important part of the diet when it comes to maintaining a healthy weight, as it passes through the body undigested and contributes very little in the way of calories. It also provides a sense of fullness to prevent overeating. Enough fiber from fruit, vegetables, pulses, legumes, and whole grains is an important component of a diet focused on weight loss.

A Balanced Plate

Balanced meals and proper portion sizes are important to liver health. But what does that mean exactly? The following section outlines the various food groups and their importance in a liver-healthy diet.

Protein

Not all protein-containing foods are the same. It's important to be aware of various types of protein-containing foods and their impact on liver health. For example, high meat consumption has been shown to be tied to NAFLD. Highly processed meat consumption is also associated with an increased risk of NAFLD, given the content of sodium, food additives, and saturated fat. In fact, Western diets are often associated with NAFLD because they tend to be higher in animal source protein, whereas diets heavy in vegetable sources are not as readily associated with NAFLD. Healthy protein-containing foods include lentils, kidney beans, and soy.

Carbohydrates

Research suggests that the type of carbohydrate consumed is a factor in liver health. Avoiding excess sugar and selecting foods that are sources of complex, rather than simple, carbohydrates is important. Fiber is a great example of a complex carbohydrate, and foods high in fiber include grain bread, beans, and asparagus.

Fats

Unsaturated fats are important to liver health because they prevent accumulation of fat in the liver, whereas saturated fats consumed in excess have been shown to increase fat. Eating a diet full of foods rich in unsaturated fats like nuts, beans, avocadoes, and olive oil has been known to have beneficial effects on NAFLD.

Vitamins and Minerals

Consuming vitamins and minerals in adequate amounts is an important part of liver and general health. Patients with NAFLD may have decreased levels of zinc, copper, carotenoids, and vitamins A, C, D, and E. Consuming a variety of foods rich in these nutrients may help ensure adequate intake. Examples of micronutrient-rich foods include carrots, papaya, and almonds.

Beverages

Sugar-filled beverages like soda are detrimental to liver health. These high-fructose corn syrup (HFCS) drinks are mostly metabolized in the liver and are the fuel for the synthesis of fatty acids. Beverages that are better to drink include water and green tea.

PORTION CONTROL

Being aware of portion sizes for common foods can be helpful and eye-opening. Here are some portion-size guidelines to keep in mind:

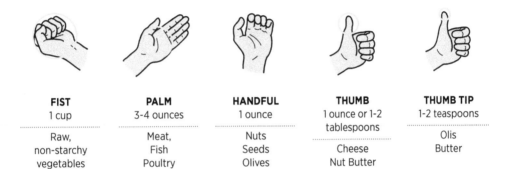

FIST	PALM	HANDFUL	THUMB	THUMB TIP
1 cup	3-4 ounces	1 ounce	1 ounce or 1-2 tablespoons	1-2 teaspoons
Raw, non-starchy vegetables	Meat, Fish Poultry	Nuts Seeds Olives	Cheese Nut Butter	Olis Butter

Watching portion sizes is really important, as it raises one's awareness of how many calories are being eaten compared with what is being burned each day. Foods such as red meat and sweetened beverages should be eaten sparingly, and being conscious of the amount is key.

MyPlate.gov is a great tool for understanding portion control. This resource provides examples of what constitutes a proper serving size of each food group. Surprisingly, a serving size of meat is about the same size as a deck of cards.

When getting started in understanding portion control, it is helpful to use measuring cups. This is relatively easy to do and can be an eye-opening exercise, especially when comparing recommended serving sizes with typical serving sizes. Plus, having this visual helps when eating at a restaurant because it will become second nature to know the proper amount to eat. You can also refer to the helpful chart above. With this awareness and knowledge, a real impact can be made on liver health.

Determining Caloric Intake and Food Servings

People often ask me what the proper number of calories is to eat in a day and what combination of foods to eat to meet that number. This section outlines appropriate caloric intake levels, how to manage to individual needs, and serving sizes of the various food types. Keep this chart handy because it's a great visual tool to assist in day-to-day caloric goals.

Daily Caloric Intake

In its purest form, weight loss happens when more energy is burned than consumed. Caloric intake plays an important role in weight loss, but the quality of the foods providing the calories is equally important. If weight loss is a goal, knowing the daily caloric adjustments to make is important. For example, to lose one pound a week, 500 fewer calories need to be consumed each day.

Daily Food Servings

The following chart provides serving guidelines for a range of daily calorie levels. Since exact calorie estimates vary widely from person to person, adjust serving sizes as outlined in the chart.

FOOD GROUP	DAILY CALORIC INTAKE			
	1,400	1,600	1,800	2,000
VEGETABLES	1½ cups	2 cups	2½ cups	2½ cups
FRUIT	1½ cups	1½ cups	1½ cups	2 cups
PROTEIN	4 ounces	5 ounces	5 ounces	5½ cups
GRAINS	5 ounces	5 ounces	6 ounces	6 ounces
DAIRY	3 cups	3 cups	3 cups	3 cups

Foods to Enjoy, Avoid, and Eat in Moderation

This section outlines what foods can be eaten freely, foods to be consumed in moderation, and foods that should be avoided. The foods listed are meant to be examples and not an exhaustive list. Stick with a diet rich in whole foods and limit processed foods high in sugar, saturated fats, and sodium.

Foods to Enjoy Freely

Fruits

- Apples
- Grapes
- Oranges

Vegetables

- Carrots
- Broccoli
- Radishes

Grains

- Brown rice
- Whole-grain bread

Proteins

- Beans
- Fish
- Walnuts

Dairy

- Low-fat or fat-free milk
- Low-fat or fat-free yogurt

Other

- Olive oil

Foods to Eat in Moderation

Proteins

- Red meat

Dairy

- Cheese
- Whole milk

Foods to Avoid

- Alcoholic beverages
- Cake
- Fried foods
- Processed meat
- Sugary snacks
- Sugar-sweetened beverages

Comorbidities and Complications

There are several complications and comorbidities related to liver disease, which we'll look at individually in this section. Depending on the issue, it may be necessary to adjust this book's advice based on individual needs.

Type 2 Diabetes

There is no one-size-fits-all eating plan for the prevention or management of diabetes, which is why it's important for adults with type 2 diabetes to receive diabetes-focused medical nutrition therapy. A key recommendation is to eat the daily recommended amount of fiber by eating plenty of fruit, vegetables, whole grains, and legumes. Other recommendations include emphasizing non-starchy vegetables, minimizing added sugars and refined grains, and choosing whole foods over highly processed foods.

Hepatitis C

The recommended diet for someone with hepatitis C is a balanced, healthy diet. It is also recommended that alcohol be avoided to prevent further liver damage. Iron may also need to be limited.

Cirrhosis

Cirrhosis of the liver can lead to malnutrition, so it's important to eat regularly, prevent muscle loss, and take the necessary steps to strengthen the muscles. Recommendations include eating four to six times per day or every one to two hours, adding protein to the diet in the form of dairy, eggs, and beans, and eating foods high in fiber, such as vegetables and whole grains. In addition, limiting salt to less than 2,000 milligrams per day may be necessary if water retention is high. Also consider eating a snack before bedtime, eating first thing in the morning, choosing dairy or fortified soy products to meet protein needs, and taking high-calorie/high-protein supplements like protein bars or shakes. Other examples of protein-containing foods to choose include nuts or nut butters, chicken, turkey, and fish. At least five servings of vegetables each day is suggested. If not enough calories or protein are being consumed, restricting salt intake is less of a concern.

Cardiovascular Disease

One of the common cardiac complications associated with NAFLD is coronary artery disease. Nutritional recommendations for coronary artery disease include reducing intake of cholesterol-raising nutrients (i.e., saturated fatty acids, *trans* fatty acids, and cholesterol), consuming additional soluble fiber and plant sterols or stanols, and balancing energy intake to maintain a healthy weight.

Sleep Apnea

Weight loss can help with sleep apnea because it reduces fatty deposits in the neck and tongue, which will help airflow. Also, weight loss reduces abdominal fat, which helps improve airflow in the lungs. Researchers believe that lower-carbohydrate diets and diets rich in fruits, vegetables, whole grains, nuts, and olive oil have therapeutic benefits for sleep apnea as well.

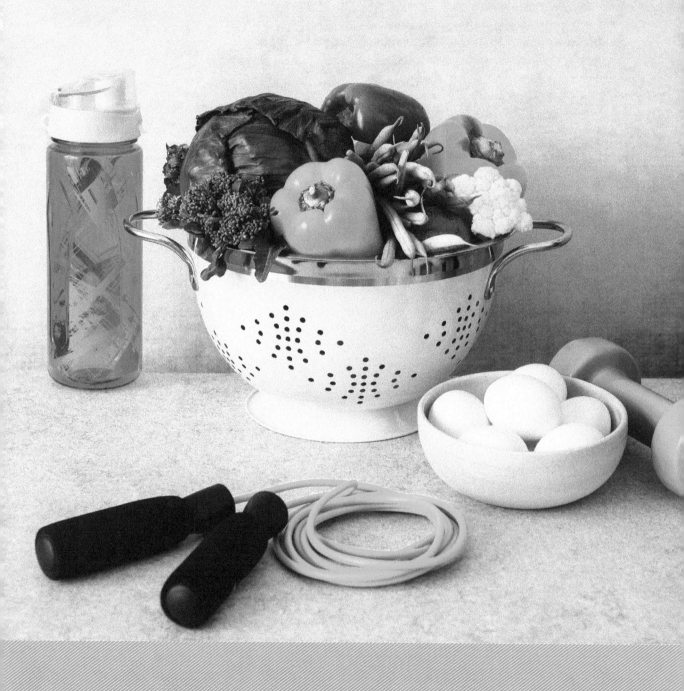

CHAPTER 2

Beyond Diet: Exercise, Toxins, and Habits

This chapter will cover the importance of exercise and liver health, as well as environmental toxins and how they affect the liver. It will also touch on sleep, stress, and healthy habits as they relate to weight loss. Finally, it will provide tips for success on sticking to the plan and how to maintain the weight loss over time.

Exercise

Exercise is a key part of losing weight and maintaining liver health. The meal plans in chapter 3 include specific daily exercise routines in addition to meals. This section discusses the various types of exercises that are important for health.

Cardiovascular Exercise (Cardio)

Cardiovascular exercise, or "cardio," increases the heart rate, improves cardiorespiratory fitness, and reduces fat in the liver. It also helps with maintaining a healthy weight, as well as brain health (with age), healthy skin, and sexual function. Moderate-intensity exercises that will increase heart rate include brisk walking, dancing, tennis, and biking.

Strength Training

Strength training, or resistance exercise, involves activities that improve muscle strength. Some studies have shown that strength training combined with cardiovascular exercise has led to weight loss and a decrease in liver fat. Strength training has also been known to improve fat breakdown and help control sugar levels in the liver. Strength training may be better for some people over cardiovascular exercise because of its lower cardiorespiratory demand, making it more accessible. In addition, strength training increases muscle mass, which leads to more calories being burned at rest. Examples of strength training include using free weights, weighted balls, or weight machines to work different muscle groups.

Stretching

Flexibility is needed to maintain joint health because it improves joint movement. Lack of flexibility can cause muscle fatigue and place stress on tissues, resulting in muscle injury at other locations besides the site of inflexibility. For example, tendonitis in the knee can be related to calf tightness. Stretching for 20 minutes several times a week outside of a training session is beneficial. The benefits of a regular stretching routine include enhanced physical performance, decreased risk of injury, and increased blood supply to joints.

Injury Prevention

Proper precautions must be taken to prevent injury during exercise. According to the American Academy of Orthopedic Surgeons, one component of safe exercise is the use of proper equipment. For example, it's important to replace shoes as they wear out and always wear comfortable clothing. Another consideration is to develop an exercise program that incorporates a variety of types; for example, cardiovascular exercise, strength training, and flexibility.

Stretching is an important component of safe exercise, and it is suggested to hold each stretch for 10 to 20 seconds to be most effective. Some research has demonstrated that warming up may help in preventing injury as well. Also be sure to drink enough water to prevent dehydration and remember to keep drinking even during exercise. Having a drink of water every 20 minutes or so can help hydration levels. Adequate rest between training sessions is also an important part of injury prevention.

Environmental Toxins

Environmental toxins are substances that negatively affect health. They include poisonous chemicals, chemical compounds, and physical materials that disrupt biological processes. It's believed that environmental toxins play a role in liver health because evidence of toxin exposure has been seen in geographical areas where many people have liver disease. Specifically, environmental toxins are thought to play major roles in the etiology and progression of NALFD. Exposure to environmental toxins has also been connected with obesity and weight increase. Specific toxin groups to be aware of include the following.

Household Products

Some fragrances, essential oils, paints, polishes, chemicals used in hair products, and other chemicals used in the home have been linked to fatty liver disease. There is still more research needed in this area to understand the full list of toxic chemicals and their lasting impact on the body.

Medications

Different types of medication have been associated with causing liver damage. However, drug-induced liver injury (DILI) occurs in a small number of people exposed to drugs, herbs, or dietary supplements and is not as common as other liver disorders. Some examples of medications that may cause liver damage are vitamin A, nonsteroidal anti-inflammatory drugs (NSAIDs), and glucocorticoids. Drugs may promote the buildup of fat in the liver as well as inflammation and fibrosis. DILI might have serious consequences like life-threatening liver failure, death, or need for liver transplantation. When taking any medication, it's important to follow the dosage amounts.

Pesticides

Pesticides are suspected to contribute to NAFLD by negatively impacting fat metabolism. Additional studies are needed in this area because it has been difficult to determine the impact on humans since many of the studies have been completed on animals. Buying organic foods as much as possible is one way to avoid exposure to pesticides.

AVOIDING TOXINS IN FOOD

Given the association between pesticides and liver disease, it's important to minimize or avoid exposure. One way to do this is to properly wash produce before cooking or consuming by gently rubbing the food under running water. There is no need to use soap or any other type of wash. For firm produce, use a clean vegetable brush to scrub off any dirt and bacteria. Rinse products before peeling to avoid the transfer of dirt and bacteria from the knife onto the produce. Drying produce with a clean cloth can also help reduce residual bacteria that may be on the surface. Handwashing before and after preparing produce is also important.

A second way to minimize toxins on food is to buy organic foods. Organic versions of many types of foods exist, including produce, grains, and meats. To cut costs, consider buying in bulk or from the freezer section. Using frozen food may be less expensive but it's also a cost savings because it helps reduce waste. Another way to cut costs is to be on the lookout for slightly blemished or oddly shaped organic produce being sold at a discount.

Sleep

Sleep is important for weight loss, and not sleeping enough may have adverse effects. The recommended number of hours to sleep a night is at least seven. Sleeping fewer than seven hours per night regularly is associated with health problems such as obesity, high blood pressure, heart disease, depression, and increased risk of death. The following steps are a great way to help get better sleep:

Remove electronics one hour before bed. The blue light coming from screens may make it more challenging to fall and stay asleep. A book is an ideal alternative to an electronic device as a way to wind down before bed.

Decrease light exposure close to bedtime. A lot of light in any sleeping environment close to bedtime may make it harder to fall asleep. Consider turning the lights down close to bedtime to prepare for sleep. Try using window shades to make the room darker if there is a lot of light coming from outside.

Get enough physical activity during the day. Being active can help with sleep. It is recommended not to exercise too close to bedtime, however. Leaving enough time between exercise and bedtime allows for body temperature and endorphin levels to return to levels that are conducive to sleep.

Sleep on a consistent schedule. Going to bed and waking up around the same time every day can help maintain a sleep-wake cycle. This means sticking to the schedule and not deviating too much on weekends.

Limit naps during the day. Sleeping too much during the day may make it difficult to fall asleep at night. Limiting the duration of naps to no more than 30 minutes can help.

Stress

Chronic stress has been associated with weight gain, impaired sleep, overeating, and the consumption of foods high in calories, like fat or sugar. To alleviate stress, it's important to move regularly and to take time for self-care. These five steps are a great way to manage stress:

Meditate for 15 minutes a day. Meditation provides an opportunity to slow down, listen, and breathe deep, all of which are good for both mental and physical health. It may be done silently or through a guided meditation.

Regular physical activity. Focusing on the body's movements can help shift away from stressful thoughts or events. Exercise can also help improve sleep, which is an important part of stress management as well. Incorporating cardio, strength training, and flexibility exercises is important when planning to be more active.

Engage with a support network. Having a support network is helpful when it comes to managing life's events. Friends and family may be able to help you take action and move forward. Being ready to navigate a complex situation is important; this might involve gathering resources in advance or bringing in others to help as needed.

Meet with a therapist. Therapists have techniques to assist with self-awareness and how to process unhelpful thoughts. Cognitive behavioral therapy (CBT) is one such approach as it examines the reasons behind certain thoughts and provides alternative ways of looking at situations.

Healthy Habits

Developing healthy habits is important when it comes to weight loss. Getting into a routine of making healthy choices will make it easier to do what is necessary to stay healthy. It is the routine behaviors that will determine health rather than the few instances of eating a certain food. The following behaviors will help form and maintain healthy habits:

Start slow. In the same way that no one would sign up for a marathon without training, jumping into an eating plan cold turkey won't be effective. Make small changes at first and enjoy the food. Same goes for exercise: Walk before running.

Identify food behavior. Notice eating patterns. Be sure to be hungry when eating rather than eating out of boredom or because of stress. Building awareness of eating patterns has an immediate effect and is the best method for making positive changes.

Enjoy food. Pick favorite foods or add more spice or flavoring to a meal that needs a little help. It's better to enjoy the meal than dread eating it next time. Food should be enjoyed with any diet change, and it's fine to include foods that are indulgent; just be mindful and conscious of when and how often.

Consistency is key. Dramatic results happen only with a consistent plan. By doing something over and over, a habit will form and those new behaviors will become routine.

Be prepared. Always be ready for those situations where there is little healthy food available. For example, if there is primarily fast food available around the workplace, consider packing a lunch.

HABIT TRACKER

The following chart may help you develop and keep track of good habits. To use this chart, list the habit in the Habit column and place an "x" in the days of the week where it was completed. For example, list *Meditate for 15 minutes* in the Habit column and then note which days of the week it was accomplished. Another example could be exercise. List *Exercise for 30 minutes* in the Habit column and then mark which days of the week that task was completed.

HABIT	MON	TUE	WED	THU	FRI	SAT	SUN

Tips for Success

Here are specific steps that will help with consistency and success with meal plans. With a little planning and prep time, it will be easy to shift a diet change into a new habit.

Meal Planning and Prepping

The meal plans in chapter 3 offer prep-ahead tips that will help eliminate spending a lot of time in the kitchen on a busy weeknight after work. Use the shopping lists and prep-ahead sections for improved organization and efficiency.

Start small: Spend a few hours on Sunday prepping. Batch cooking meals will go more quickly and feel less overwhelming.

Enjoy leftovers: Double a recipe and freeze half in individual portions for future meals.

Don't prep everything: If a recipe takes a small amount of time to prepare, don't prep it ahead of time, so that the meal is fresher. Prep dishes that take longer than 30 minutes.

Cooking Shortcuts

The recipes in this book offer smart shortcuts to save time (such as buying precut veggies or precooked rice). Once you're in the kitchen, there are several things you can do that can help make things move faster.

Have a go-to meal: For nights when you're not in the mood to cook, have a go-to meal that's quick and easy, such as a tuna salad or scrambled eggs and veggies.

Love the freezer: Double or triple a recipe and freeze leftovers in individual containers. Most will keep for about six months.

Precook and freeze grains: Precook grains such as rice or quinoa and freeze them in 1-cup amounts in zip-top bags for up to six months.

Eating Out

When eating out, it's important to check the menu carefully to avoid foods that may have a lot of added fat, sugar, and salt. Focus on whole-food items, such as fruits and vegetables, whole grains, and legumes. Make healthy substitutions, such as asking for avocado on a sandwich instead of bacon.

After the 28-Day Plan

When planning to make big diet changes, start gradually and take the time to make it natural and part of the daily routine. This typically leads to longer-term consistency and success. Remember it's important to develop healthy eating habits rather than eating a healthy meal on occasion. When eating foods not included in the diet, be mindful and practice moderation. Find healthy substitutions for unhealthy foods. For example, if cookies are on the brain, experiment with recipes that include fiber-rich flour and are naturally sweetened with ingredients like dates.

Maintaining long-term weight loss is about consistency and forming good habits. Enjoyment of food is always key to a sustainable diet, so be sure to add variety to keep things interesting and tasty. Food can be creamy, sweet, and flavorful when made with healthy ingredients, so explore different options.

Adjust your diet and physical activity based on individual needs. If trying to lose weight, create a calorie deficit by burning more calories than consumed. Once your goal weight is reached, shift to a matching calorie-in/calorie-out diet to maintain weight. Keeping track of weight on a regular basis will help manage needs. It's important to remember that eating well for liver health can be customized to suit individual preferences and needs, and there is a range of food options that fit within the recommendations. Experiment with food and make it fun!

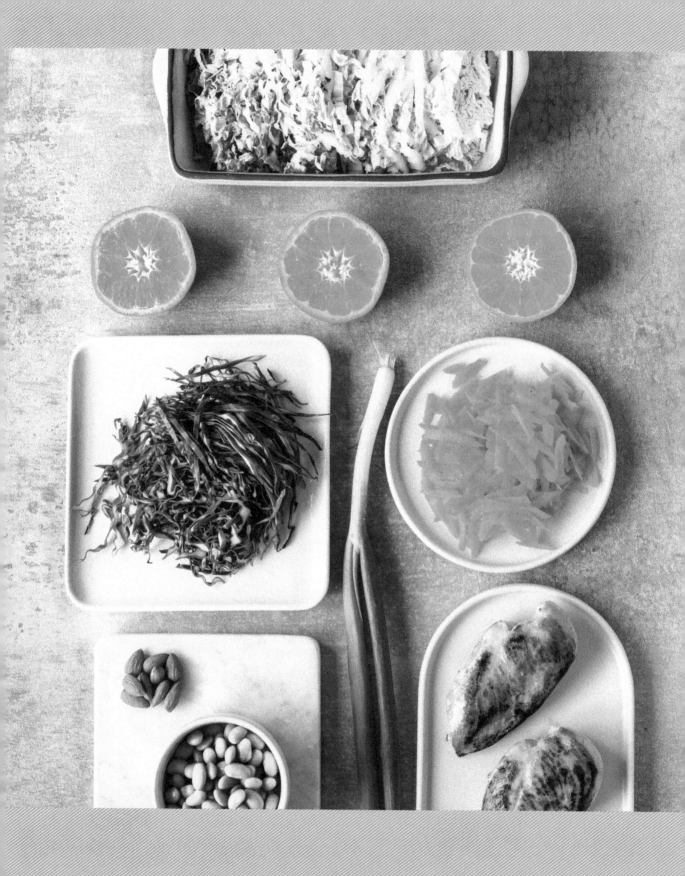

CHAPTER 3

The 28-Day Weight Loss Plan

A meal plan filled with nutritious, unprocessed whole foods means making food from scratch. If processed, manufactured, or premade foods have been the plan in the past, kitchen time will probably increase, but that doesn't mean less free time. These meal plans and recipes are designed to be quick and easy using simple, affordable, and easy-to-find ingredients. Although most recipes make more than one serving, they're intended for a single person using leftovers as future lunches or dinners. Recipes also save time with quick or make-ahead breakfasts, easy lunches, and fast weeknight meals.

Feeding More

Interested in feeding more than one person with some of the meals in the meal plans? Recipes can easily be doubled and tripled to feed the whole family or a group of friends.

Making Substitutions

The meal plans are a guideline. If an ingredient isn't available or something doesn't sound tasty, be flexible! Substitute any main dish recipe for any other in this cookbook. Likewise, substitute fish, shellfish, white-meat poultry, or minimally processed plant-based proteins for main dishes. Replace herbs, spices, fruits, or vegetables for a different ingredient in the same category.

Please remember that it is always important to consult with a doctor before starting any diet change or weight-loss plan.

WEEK 1

	BREAKFAST	LUNCH	SNACK	DINNER	EXERCISE
MON	Apple Cinnamon Overnight Oats (page 47)	Whole-Wheat Pita Chips (page 121) with Hummus and Bell Peppers (page 118)	Apple plus 2 tablespoons peanut butter	Turkey Tapenade Burgers (page 107)	Cardio (page 135) Upper Body (page 136)
TUE	*Leftover Apple Cinnamon Overnight Oats*	*Leftover Turkey Tapenade Burgers*	*Leftover Hummus and Bell Peppers*	Whole-Wheat Pasta Puttanesca (page 74)	Cardio (page 135) Core (page 136)
WED	*Leftover Apple Cinnamon Overnight Oats*	*Leftover Turkey Tapenade Burgers*	*Leftover Hummus and Bell Peppers*	*Leftover Whole-Wheat Pasta Puttanesca*	Cardio (page 135) Lower Body (page 136)
THU	*Leftover Apple Cinnamon Overnight Oats*	*Leftover Turkey Tapenade Burgers*	*Leftover Hummus and Bell Peppers*	Butternut Squash Soup with Pepitas (page 76)	Rest day
FRI	Avo-Egg Toast (page 54)	*Leftover Whole-Wheat Pasta Puttanesca*	Apple plus 2 tablespoons peanut butter	*Leftover Butternut Squash Soup with Pepitas*	Cardio (page 135)
SAT	*Leftover Avo-Egg Toast*	*Leftover Whole-Wheat Pasta Puttanesca*	Lemon-Garlic Kale Chips (page 116)	Baked Turkey Kofta Meatballs with Tricolored Peppers (page 104)	Full Body (page 136) Cardio (page 135)
SUN	Spinach Egg Muffins (page 52)	*Leftover Butternut Squash Soup with Pepitas*	2 carrots plus 2 tablespoons peanut butter	Southwestern Black Bean Chili (page 77)	Rest day

Shopping List

PRODUCE

- ☐ Apples (2)
- ☐ Arugula (1 bunch)
- ☐ Avocado (1)
- ☐ Basil, fresh (1 bunch)
- ☐ Bell peppers, any color (5)
- ☐ Bell pepper, green (1)
- ☐ Butternut squash (1)
- ☐ Carrots (2)
- ☐ Garlic (2 bulbs)
- ☐ Ginger (1)
- ☐ Kale (16 ounces)
- ☐ Lemon (3)
- ☐ Onion, small red (1)
- ☐ Onion, yellow (3)
- ☐ Parsley (1 bunch)
- ☐ Spinach, baby (9-ounce bag)
- ☐ Tomato, small (1)

DAIRY AND EGGS

- ☐ Cheese, low-fat Cheddar (2 ounces)
- ☐ Eggs (18)
- ☐ Milk (½ gallon)

MEAT AND SEAFOOD

- ☐ Ground turkey breast (2 pounds)

PANTRY

- ☐ Allspice, ground
- ☐ Beans, black (2 [14-ounce] cans)
- ☐ Black peppercorns
- ☐ Capers (1 jar)
- ☐ Chia seeds
- ☐ Chickpeas (1 [14-ounce] can)
- ☐ Chili powder
- ☐ Cinnamon, ground
- ☐ Coriander, ground
- ☐ Cumin, ground
- ☐ Garlic powder
- ☐ Ginger, ground
- ☐ Italian seasoning
- ☐ Mustard, Dijon
- ☐ Nonstick cooking spray
- ☐ Oats, old-fashioned rolled
- ☐ Oil, olive
- ☐ Olives, black (1 [4-ounce] can)
- ☐ Oregano, dried
- ☐ Paprika, ground
- ☐ Peanut butter
- ☐ Pepitas
- ☐ Red pepper flakes, dried
- ☐ Sage, ground
- ☐ Salt, sea
- ☐ Spaghetti, whole-wheat (8 ounces)

Tahini

Tomatoes, diced (2 [28-ounce] cans)

Vegetable broth, low-sodium
(32 ounces)

Vinegar, red wine

Walnuts

OTHER

Apples, dried (¾ cup)

Bread, whole-wheat
(freeze leftovers)

Pita bread, whole-wheat
(freeze leftovers)

Prep Ahead

Prep this week is relatively light and can easily be done on Sunday.

- If making the vegetable broth from scratch, make it on Sunday, and store, tightly sealed, in the refrigerator.
- Prepare the oats overnight and refrigerate.
- Make hummus and store, tightly sealed, in the refrigerator.
- Make tapenade and store, tightly sealed, in the refrigerator.
- Cut bell peppers and store in the refrigerator for the Baked Turkey Kofta Meatballs with Tricolored Peppers (page 104).
- Peel and cut butternut squash and store, tightly sealed, in the refrigerator.
- Chop bell peppers and onions for the Southwestern Black Bean Chili (page 77) and store in the refrigerator.

WEEK 2

	BREAKFAST	LUNCH	SNACK	DINNER	EXERCISE
MON	*Leftover Spinach Egg Muffins*	*Leftover Butternut Squash Soup with Pepitas*	*Leftover Lemon-Garlic Kale chips*	*Leftover Baked Turkey Kofta Meatballs with Tricolored Peppers*	Cardio (page 135) Upper Body (page 136)
TUE	Greek Yogurt Bowls with Berries (page 46)	*Leftover Baked Turkey Kofta Meatballs with Tricolored Peppers*	½ avocado plus 2 tablespoons pepitas	Weeknight Cioppino (page 88)	Cardio (page 135) Core (page 136)
WED	*Leftover Spinach Egg Muffins*	*Leftover Baked Turkey Kofta Meatballs with Tricolored Peppers*	*Leftover Lemon-Garlic Kale chips*	*Leftover Weeknight Cioppino*	Cardio (page 135) Lower Body (page 136)
THU	*Leftover Greek Yogurt Bowls with Berries*	*Leftover Southwestern Black Bean Chili*	½ avocado plus 2 tablespoons pepitas	Lentil Curry (page 80)	Rest day
FRI	Pumpkin Pie Smoothie (page 48)	*Leftover Southwestern Black Bean Chili*	2 carrots plus 2 tablespoons peanut butter	*Leftover Lentil Curry*	Cardio (page 135)
SAT	Buckwheat Pancakes with Fruit Compote (page 49)	*Leftover Weeknight Cioppino*	Orange-Cranberry Compote (page 133)	Patty Melt Soup (page 110)	Cardio (page 135) Full Body (page 136)
SUN	Bell Pepper and Feta Frittata (page 50)	*Leftover Weeknight Cioppino*	2 hard-boiled eggs	Spice-Rubbed Crispy Roast Chicken (page 100)	Rest day

Shopping List

PRODUCE

Avocado (1)

Bell pepper, orange (1)

Bell pepper, red (2)

Blackberries (1 pint)

Blueberries (1 pint)

Carrots (5)

Garlic (1 bulb)

Onion, yellow (5)

Orange (1)

Parsley (1 bunch)

Raspberries (1 pint)

Strawberries (1 pint)

Sweet potatoes (2)

DAIRY AND EGGS

Eggs (1 dozen)

Feta cheese (4 ounces)

Greek yogurt, plain (8 ounces)

MEAT AND SEAFOOD

Beef, ground, extra-lean (1 pound)

Chicken legs (6)

Cod, skinless (8 ounces)

Shrimp, medium, tail off and peeled (8 ounces)

FROZEN

Cranberries (12-ounce bag frozen or fresh)

PANTRY

Baking powder

Buckwheat flour

Caraway seeds, ground

Cayenne

Curry powder

Honey

Lentils (2 [14-ounce] cans)

Maple syrup, pure

Mustard powder

Pumpkin pie spice

Pumpkin puree (1 [15-ounce] can)

Tomatoes, diced (1 [14-ounce] can)

Tomato sauce (1 [14-ounce] can)

Vanilla extract

Vegetable broth, low-sodium (96 ounces)

Prep Ahead

This is a super-low prep week and involves only chopping vegetables.

- If making the vegetable broth from scratch, make it on Sunday, and store, tightly sealed, in the refrigerator.
- Chop an onion and red bell pepper for the Weeknight Cioppino (page 88) and store together in a zip-top bag in the refrigerator.
- Chop the onions and sweet potatoes for the Lentil Curry (page 80) and store in a zip-top bag in the refrigerator.
- Slice onions for the Patty Melt Soup (page 110) and store in a zip-top bag in the refrigerator.

WEEK 3

	BREAKFAST	LUNCH	SNACK	DINNER	EXERCISE
MON	*Leftover Pumpkin Pie Smoothie*	Chicken Chopped Salad (page 62)	2 hard-boiled eggs	*Leftover Spice-Rubbed Crispy Roast Chicken*	Cardio (page 135) Upper Body (page 136)
TUE	*Leftover Buckwheat Pancakes with Fruit Compote*	*Leftover Chicken Chopped Salad*	2 hard-boiled eggs	*Leftover Patty Melt Soup*	Cardio (page 135) Core (page 136)
WED	*Leftover Spinach Egg Muffins*	Leftover Chicken Chopped Salad	Apple-Ginger Slaw (page 64)	*Leftover Lentil Curry*	Cardio (page 135) Lower Body (page 136)
THU	*Leftover Bell Pepper Feta Frittata*	*Leftover Chicken Chopped Salad*	*Leftover Apple-Ginger Slaw*	Shrimp Fried Cauliflower Rice (page 91)	Rest day
FRI	*Leftover Spinach Egg Muffins*	*Leftover Southwestern Black Bean Chili*	*Leftover Apple-Ginger Slaw*	*Leftover Patty Melt Soup*	Cardio (page 135)
SAT	Shakshuka (page 44)	*Leftover Shrimp Cauliflower Fried Rice*	*Leftover Apple-Ginger Slaw*	Mediterranean Chicken Skillet (page 106)	Cardio (page 135) Full Body (page 136)
SUN	*Leftover Shakshuka*	*Leftover Mediterranean Chicken Skillet*	Ponzu Grilled Avocado (page 65)	Pesto-Stuffed Chicken Roulade (page 108)	Rest Day

Shopping List

PRODUCE

- Apples (4)
- Avocado (2)
- Basil (1 bunch)
- Bell pepper, red (5)
- Carrot (1)
- Cauliflower (1 head)
- Fennel (1 bulb)
- Garlic (1 bulb)
- Ginger
- Lemon (3)
- Lime (1)
- Lettuce, romaine (1 head)
- Onion, red (1)
- Onion, yellow (1)
- Parsley (1 bunch)
- Scallions (2 bunches)
- Spinach, baby (1 [9-ounce] bag)
- Tomatoes, cherry (1 pint)
- Tomatoes, Roma (2)
- Zucchini, medium (1)

DAIRY AND EGGS

- Cheese, Parmesan (4 ounces)
- Eggs (1 dozen)
- Yogurt, Greek (16 ounces)

MEAT AND SEAFOOD

- Chicken breast, boneless and skinless (2 pounds)
- Shrimp, medium, tail off and peeled (1 pound)

PANTRY

- Artichoke hearts, (1 [14-ounce] can)
- Chickpeas, no salt (1 [15-ounce] can)
- Crushed tomatoes, no salt (1 [28-ounce] can)
- Olives, sliced (1 [4-ounce] can)
- Paprika, smoked
- Pine nuts
- Sesame seeds
- Soy sauce or tamari, low-sodium
- Vinegar, apple cider
- Vinegar, red wine
- Vinegar, rice

Prep Ahead

- Hard-boil six eggs for snacks. Store in the refrigerator.
- Chop the onion and bell peppers for the Shakshuka (page 44) and store in the refrigerator.
- Chop the zucchini and scallions and make the Greek Lemon Vinaigrette (page 126) for the Chicken Chopped Salad (page 62).
- Chop the red onion for the Mediterranean Chicken Skillet (page 106) and store in the refrigerator.
- Chop the vegetables and grate the cauliflower for the Shrimp Fried Cauliflower Rice (page 91) and refrigerate.

WEEK 4

	BREAKFAST	LUNCH	SNACK	DINNER	EXERCISE
MON	*Leftover Shakshuka*	*Leftover Shrimp Cauliflower Fried Rice*	*Leftover Ponzu Grilled Avocado*	*Leftover Mediterranean Chicken Skillet*	Cardio (page 135) Upper Body (page 136)
TUE	*Leftover Shakshuka*	*Leftover Patty Melt Soup*	*Leftover Ponzu Grilled Avocado*	*Leftover Pesto-Stuffed Chicken Roulade*	Cardio (page 135) Core (page 136)
WED	*Leftover Bell Pepper Feta Frittata*	*Leftover Lentil Curry*	*Leftover Ponzu Grilled Avocado*	*Leftover Southwestern Black Bean chili*	Cardio (page 135) Lower Body (page 136)
THU	*Leftover Spinach Egg Muffins*	*Leftover Patty Melt Soup*	*Leftover Cranberry-Orange Compote*	Ground Turkey and Veggie Stir-Fry (page 105)	Rest day
FRI	*Leftover Bell Pepper Feta Frittata*	*Leftover Shrimp Cauliflower Fried Rice*	*Leftover Cranberry-Orange Compote*	*Leftover Ground Turkey and Veggie Stir-Fry*	Cardio (page 135)
SAT	Avo-Egg Toast (page 54)	*Leftover Shrimp Cauliflower Fried Rice*	Baba Ghanoush and Veggies (page 117)	*Leftover Patty Melt Soup*	Cardio (page 135) Full Body (page 136)
SUN	*Leftover Avo-Egg Toast*	*Leftover Ground Turkey and Veggie Stir-Fry*	*Leftover Cranberry-Orange Compote*	Mustard and Herb Pork Tenderloin (page 109)	Rest day

Shopping List

PRODUCE

- Avocado (1)
- Bell pepper, red (1)
- Broccoli (2 bunches)
- Carrots (12)
- Eggplant (2)
- Garlic (1 bulb)
- Lemon (1)
- Onions, red (2)
- Orange (1)
- Parsley (1 bunch)
- Potatoes, baby red (1 pound)
- Rosemary, fresh (1 bunch)
- Scallions (1 bunch)

MEAT AND SEAFOOD

- Pork tenderloin (1 pound)
- Turkey breast, ground (1 pound)

PANTRY

- Brown rice, cooked

Prep Ahead

There are lots of leftovers this week from both the refrigerator and freezer, so food prep is light during this final week of the plan.

- Cook the brown rice and store in 1-cup servings in the refrigerator or freezer.
- Chop the carrots, scallions, broccoli, and bell pepper for the Ground Turkey and Veggie Stir-Fry (page 105) and refrigerate.

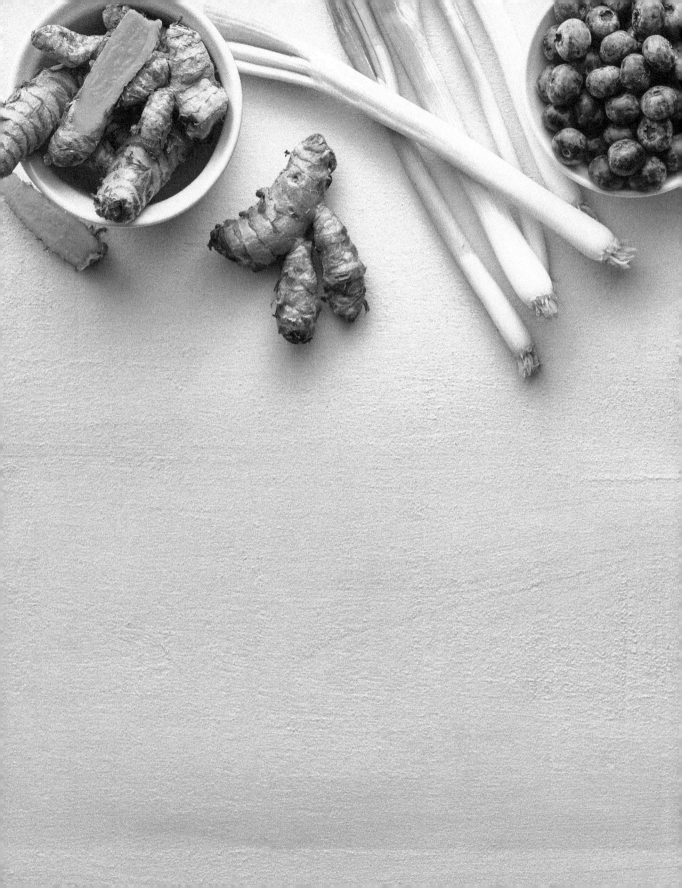

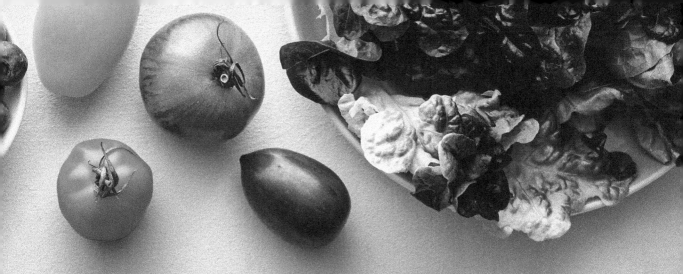

PART TWO

THE RECIPES

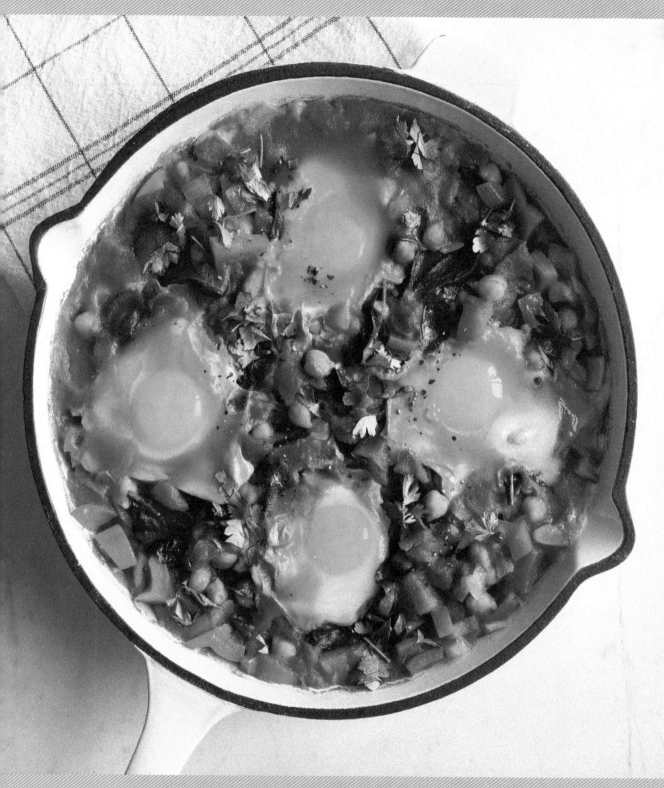

Shakshuka, page 44.

CHAPTER 4

Breakfast and Beverages

Shakshuka

Prep time: 10 minutes | **Cook time:** 20 minutes | Makes 4

This traditional Middle Eastern dish has become trendy at brunch spots, but it's super easy to make at home. It's loaded with delicious, aromatic spices in a hearty tomato sauce that's as nutritious as it is delicious. If feeling adventurous, experiment with a personal spice blend. Good add-ins include ground coriander, cinnamon, and nutmeg.

2 tablespoons extra-virgin olive oil

1 red bell pepper, seeded, ribs removed, and chopped

½ large yellow onion, chopped

1 (28-ounce) can no-salt-added crushed tomatoes

1 (15-ounce) can no-salt added chickpeas, drained and rinsed

2 teaspoons ground cumin

2 teaspoons ground smoked paprika

1 teaspoon garlic powder

½ teaspoon freshly ground black pepper

4 large eggs

¼ cup coarsely chopped fresh parsley

1. In a large skillet, heat the olive oil over medium heat. Add the bell pepper and onion and cook for 3 minutes, or until the onion becomes translucent.

2. Stir in the tomatoes with their juices, chickpeas, cumin, smoked paprika, garlic powder, and black pepper to combine. Cook for 10 minutes, stirring occasionally.

3. With the back of a spoon, create four wells in the tomato sauce. Gently crack 1 egg into each well. Cover the skillet and cook for 7 minutes, or until the egg whites are set. Remove from the heat. Top the shakshuka with the parsley.

4. This is best eaten fresh; however, if needed, store in the refrigerator in single-serving containers for up to 3 days.

TIP: Add some goat cheese or feta cheese for a sharper contrast of flavors.

Per Serving (1 egg and ½ cup sauce): Calories: 310; Protein: 16g; Total fat: 14g; Total carbohydrates: 33g; Fiber: 9g; Sugars: 8g; Sodium: 445 mg; Iron: 5mg

Sweet Potato, Onion, and Turkey Sausage Hash

Prep time: 10 minutes | **Cook time:** 25 minutes | Makes 4

Sweet potatoes are higher in fiber (even more so when they're not peeled, as in this dish) than white potatoes, and they add an earthy sweetness that contrasts with the pungent sage and aromatic garlic in the homemade turkey sausage. Don't let the words "homemade turkey sausage" intimidate; it's super easy to make and much lower in salt than premade sausage.

1 tablespoon extra-virgin olive oil

2 medium sweet potatoes, cut into ½-inch dice

8 servings Homemade Turkey Breakfast Sausage (page 125; skip steps 2 and 3)

1 small onion, chopped

½ red bell pepper, seeded, ribs removed, and chopped

2 garlic cloves, minced

Chopped fresh parsley, for garnish

1. In a large skillet, heat the olive oil over medium-high heat. Add the sweet potatoes and cook, stirring occasionally, for 12 to 15 minutes, until they brown and begin to soften.

2. Add the turkey sausage, onion, bell pepper, and garlic. Cook for 5 to 6 minutes, until the turkey sausage is cooked through and the vegetables soften.

3. Sprinkle with parsley and serve warm.

4. Store in the refrigerator in single-serving containers for up to 3 days or freeze for up to 3 months.

TIP: Double the amount of turkey sausage. Use half with this recipe, and then cook the rest, crumbling in a pan. Store it in the freezer for use in future breakfasts. It will keep for about 6 months.

Per Serving (about ½ cup): Calories: 190; Protein: 12g; Total fat: 7g; Total carbohydrates: 16g; Fiber: 3g; Sugars: 7g; Sodium: 197mg; Iron: 2mg

Greek Yogurt Bowls with Berries

Prep time: 10 minutes | Makes 2

Greek yogurt is creamy and tangy, and it offers a balanced counterpoint to the sweetness of the berries. Although fresh or thawed frozen berries can be used (if using frozen, make sure they are sugar-free), fresh berries in season are sweeter and more satisfying. Use any combination of berries for a fast and easy no-cook breakfast.

1 cup plain Greek yogurt

¼ cup blueberries

¼ cup sliced strawberries

¼ cup blackberries

¼ cup raspberries

2 tablespoons pepitas
(pumpkin seeds)

1. Spoon the yogurt into two small bowls.

2. In a small bowl, mix the berries. Spoon an equal amount into both bowls. Stir to mix the berries and yogurt.

3. Sprinkle each bowl with 1 tablespoon of pepitas.

4. If storing the second serving, stir together the fruit and yogurt and cover. Store for up to 3 days in the refrigerator. Sprinkle with the pepitas just before eating.

TIP: This is delicious with berries, but you can try 1 cup of any chopped, soft fruits, such as peaches, plums, nectarines, or melon, for a sweet and satisfying breakfast.

Per Serving (about ½ cup of yogurt and ½ cup of berries):
Calories: 150; Protein: 7g; Total fat: 8g; Total carbohydrates: 15g;
Fiber: 3g; Sugars: 10g; Sodium: 58mg; Iron: 1mg

Apple Cinnamon Overnight Oats

Prep time: 5 minutes, plus overnight to chill | Makes 4

On Pinterest, there are overnight oats individually portioned in cute jam and jelly jars. Those are cute, but not necessary. Just mix up a batch in a bowl, refrigerate it overnight, and spoon it into any individual container in the morning. It's fast, easy, and a super-tasty way to enjoy no-cook oatmeal for breakfast.

1½ cups skim milk or low-fat unsweetened nondairy milk, such as almond milk or oat milk

1½ cups old-fashioned oats

¾ cup chopped dried apples

2 tablespoons chia seeds

1 teaspoon ground cinnamon

¼ cup chopped walnuts or pecans

1. In a medium bowl, mix the milk, oats, dried apples, chia seeds, and cinnamon.

2. Cover and refrigerate overnight.

3. Spoon into four containers and sprinkle with the walnuts.

4. Store in single-serving containers in the refrigerator for up to 5 days.

TIP: Dried cranberries also work well. Replace the apples with cranberries or opt for a combination of dried apples and dried cranberries.

Per Serving (about ¾ cup): Calories: 191; Protein: 10g; Total fat: 9g; Total carbohydrates: 29g; Fiber: 8g; Sugars: 7g; Sodium: 51mg; Iron: 2mg

Pumpkin Pie Smoothie

Prep time: 5 minutes | Makes 2

Fall isn't the only time to enjoy pumpkin spice flavors. This smoothie brings all the deliciousness of everybody's favorite Thanksgiving dessert year-round with just a quick spin in the blender. It's a tasty and nutritious way to start the day, and the aromatic spices and earthy pumpkin will wake up any palate.

2 cups skim milk or unsweetened nondairy milk, such as oat milk

1½ cups canned pumpkin puree (not pumpkin pie filling)

2 tablespoons pure maple syrup

2 tablespoons chia seeds

1 teaspoon pumpkin pie spice

½ teaspoon vanilla extract

½ cup crushed ice

1. In a blender, combine the milk, pumpkin puree, maple syrup, chia seeds, pumpkin pie spice, vanilla, and ice. Blend until smooth.

2. Pour into two containers. The second drink can be stored in the refrigerator for up to 3 days. Shake or reblend before serving.

TIP: Don't have pumpkin pie spice? No worries—make it from scratch by combining ½ teaspoon ground cinnamon, ¼ teaspoon ground ginger, 2 pinches ground nutmeg, and a pinch each of allspice and ground cloves.

Per Serving (about 1¼ cups): Calories: 276; Protein: 13g; Total fat: 5g; Total carbohydrates: 47g; Fiber: 10g; Sugars: 30g; Sodium: 143mg; Iron: 4mg

Buckwheat Pancakes with Fruit Compote

Prep time: 5 minutes | **Cook time:** 15 minutes | Makes 4

Buckwheat adds a nutty flavor and toothsome bite to pancakes. This gluten-free version has a fluffy texture that soaks up the sweet, jammy juices from the fruit compote.

2 cups mixed berries (fresh or frozen)

2 tablespoons water

½ teaspoon ground cinnamon

1½ cups buckwheat flour

1 teaspoon baking powder

1¼ cups skim milk or unsweetened nondairy milk

1 egg, beaten

1 tablespoon pure maple syrup (optional)

1 teaspoon vanilla extract

Nonstick cooking spray

1. In a small saucepan, heat the berries, water, and cinnamon over medium-high heat, stirring occasionally, until the berries are soft. Set aside.

2. In a small bowl, whisk together the buckwheat flour and baking powder.

3. In another small bowl, whisk together the milk, egg, maple syrup, and vanilla.

4. Add the wet ingredients to the dry ingredients and fold until just combined.

5. Heat a nonstick skillet over medium-high heat and spray with cooking spray.

6. Working in batches, pour the batter in scant ¼ cup measures onto the heated skillet.

7. When bubbles form on top of the pancakes (after 2 to 3 minutes), flip. Cook for another 2 to 3 minutes. Serve topped with the berry compote.

8. Store in the refrigerator for up to 4 days. Store the pancakes and compote separately.

TIP: If a sweeter compote is preferred, add 1 packet of stevia to the berries as they cook.

Per Serving (about 2 pancakes and 2 tablespoons of compote): Calories: 226; Protein: 10g; Total fat: 3g; Total carbohydrates: 43g; Fiber: 6g; Sugars: 9g; Sodium: 147mg; Iron: 3mg

Bell Pepper and Feta Frittata

Prep time: 10 minutes | **Cook time:** 15 minutes | Makes 4

For a little bit of breakfast magic in virtually no time at all, whip up this colorful and delicious frittata. It's like the pizza of the breakfast world—simply cut it into wedges and serve. Enjoy one now, then enjoy the others reheated for breakfast later in the week. And, if breakfast for dinner sounds appealing, this makes the perfect fast weeknight meal.

6 eggs, beaten

1 teaspoon Italian seasoning

½ teaspoon sea salt

¼ teaspoon freshly ground black pepper

2 tablespoons extra-virgin olive oil

½ red bell pepper, seeded, ribs removed, and sliced

½ orange bell pepper, seeded, ribs removed, and sliced

½ yellow onion, peeled and thinly sliced

1 garlic clove, minced

¼ cup crumbled feta cheese

1. Preheat the oven's broiler on high.

2. In a medium bowl, whisk together the eggs, Italian seasoning, salt, and black pepper. Set aside.

3. In a 12-inch oven-safe skillet, heat the olive oil over medium-high heat until it shimmers.

4. Add the bell peppers and onion and cook, stirring occasionally, until the vegetables are soft, about 5 minutes.

5. Add the garlic and cook, stirring constantly, for 30 seconds.

6. Spread the vegetables in an even layer on the bottom of the pan. Carefully pour the egg mixture over the top, making sure it creates an even layer over and around the vegetables.

7. Cook without stirring until the eggs begin to set, about 4 minutes.

8. Sprinkle with the feta and transfer to under the broiler. Cook until the cheese melts and the tops of the eggs set, about 3 minutes more.

9. Cut into four wedges.

10. Store remaining wedges in zip-top bags in the refrigerator for up to 3 days or freeze for up to 6 months.

TIP: A cast-iron pan is the ideal oven-safe skillet for making frittatas, if available. If not, make sure the pan has an oven-safe handle before placing it under the broiler.

Per Serving (1 wedge): Calories: 208; Protein: 11g; Total fat: 16g; Total carbohydrates: 4g; Fiber: 1g; Sugars: 3g; Sodium: 485mg; Iron: 2mg

Spinach Egg Muffins

Prep time: 15 minutes | **Cook time:** 15 minutes | Makes 6

These "muffins" are the ultimate make-ahead breakfast. They store and reheat really well, and the only limitation is how many can be made by the number of muffin tin cups available. They're delicious, packed with protein, and perfect for busy people who need a satisfying breakfast on the go.

Nonstick cooking spray (optional)

2 tablespoons extra-virgin olive oil

½ yellow onion, chopped

4 cups baby spinach

2 garlic cloves, minced

12 eggs

½ teaspoon sea salt

¼ teaspoon freshly ground black pepper

½ cup grated low-fat Cheddar cheese (optional)

1. Preheat the oven to 350°F. Spray a 6-cup muffin tin with nonstick cooking spray (or line them with silicone muffin tin liners).

2. In a large skillet, heat the olive oil over medium-high heat until it shimmers.

3. Add the onion and cook, stirring occasionally, until soft, 3 to 4 minutes.

4. Add the spinach and cook until it softens, about 3 minutes more.

5. Add the garlic and cook, stirring constantly, for 30 seconds.

6. Remove the vegetables from the heat and set aside to let cool.

7. In a large bowl, whisk together the eggs, salt, and pepper.

8. Fold in the cooled vegetables and cheese (if using).

9. Spoon into the prepared muffin tin.

10. Bake in the oven until the eggs set, about 15 minutes.

11. Store remaining cooled muffins in individual zip-top bags in the refrigerator for up to 3 days or freeze for up to 6 months.

TIP: Silicone muffin tin liners are the perfect accessory for making these; they are reusable and eliminate the need for cooking spray.

Per Serving (1 muffin): Calories: 193; Protein: 13g; Total fat: 14g; Total carbohydrates: 3g; Fiber: 1g; Sugars: 1g; Sodium: 255mg; Iron: 2mg

Avo-Egg Toast

Prep time: 10 minutes | **Cook time:** 5 minutes | Makes 2

Avocado toast is popular for a good reason—it's delicious, and it's packed with fiber and lots of vitamins and minerals. Adding an egg on top adds more flavor and some protein, creating a stick-to-the-ribs breakfast that's ready fast. Try a high-fiber bread such as whole wheat, Ezekiel bread, or a favorite gluten-free bread.

½ avocado, peeled, pitted, and mashed with a fork

1 teaspoon freshly squeezed lemon juice

½ teaspoon sea salt, divided

2 slices whole-grain bread, toasted

1 tablespoon extra-virgin olive oil

2 eggs

2 tablespoons pepitas

¼ teaspoon freshly ground black pepper

1. In a small bowl, mix the avocado, lemon juice, and ¼ teaspoon of salt.

2. Spread on the slices of toast.

3. In a medium nonstick skillet, heat the olive oil over low heat until it is warm.

4. Crack the eggs carefully into the pan. Cook without stirring until the whites set.

5. Turn off the heat and carefully flip the eggs. Allow to sit for 30 to 60 seconds to slightly cook the yolks.

6. Top each slice of toast with an egg. Sprinkle with the pepitas and season with the pepper.

7. These really don't store well; it's best to cook to order since they are so quick to make.

TIP: The method here calls for over-easy eggs. If yolks with a harder set are preferred, then leave the heat on when flipping the eggs. They will set in about 2 minutes.

Per Serving (1 toast and 1 egg): Calories: 324; Protein: 13g; Total fat: 24g; Total carbohydrates: 17g; Fiber: 6g; Sugars: 2g; Sodium: 389mg; Iron: 2mg

Breakfast Scramble Pitas

Prep time: 5 minutes | **Cook time:** 10 minutes | Makes 4

Pita pockets are a convenient way to eat breakfast on the go. These convenient breakfast sandwiches are flavorful and oh-so satisfying. With protein from the eggs and fiber from whole-grain pitas, they'll satisfy for hours and help prevent the mid-morning slump.

2 whole-wheat pitas, split in half

½ avocado, peeled, pitted, and mashed with a fork

1 tablespoon canola oil

6 eggs, beaten

½ teaspoon sea salt

¼ teaspoon freshly ground black pepper

½ cup cherry tomatoes, halved

6 fresh basil leaves, cut into strips

1. Open each pita half and spread with the mashed avocado.

2. In a medium nonstick skillet, heat the canola oil over low heat until it is warm.

3. Add the eggs, salt, and pepper. Cook, scrambling, until the eggs are set, about 4 minutes.

4. Remove from the heat and add the cherry tomatoes and fresh basil. Stir to mix.

5. Spoon into the prepared pitas.

6. Store the eggs, pitas, mashed avocado, and tomatoes/basil separately in the refrigerator for up to 3 days. Do not freeze. Reheat the eggs and assemble the sandwiches to serve.

TIP: To store mashed avocado, put it in a small bowl, squeeze a little lemon juice over the top, and then put plastic wrap directly on the surface of the avocado to keep the air out. This will keep the avocado from browning. Store for up to 3 days.

Per Serving (1 pita): Calories: 264; Protein: 13g; Total fat: 15g; Total carbohydrates: 20g; Fiber: 3g; Sugars: 1g; Sodium: 415mg; Iron: 2mg

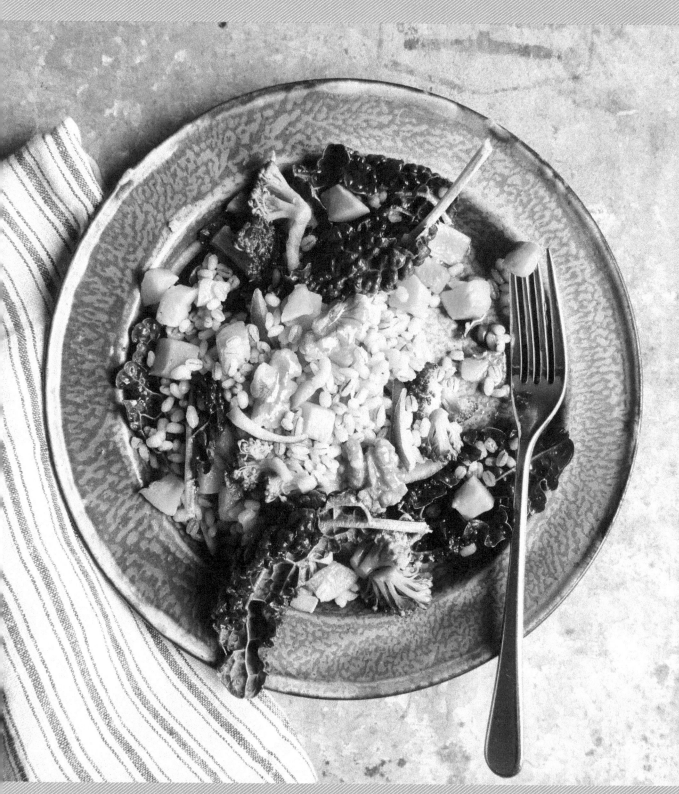

Warm Barley and Squash Salad with Balsamic Vinaigrette, page 58.

CHAPTER 5

Sides and Salads

Warm Barley and Squash Salad with Balsamic Vinaigrette

Prep time: 20 minutes | **Cook time:** 40 minutes | Makes 8

Butternut squash is easy to prepare and has a naturally sweet, creamy taste that works well in so many dishes. Packed with vitamins A and C, squash even has anticancer properties that make it a valuable addition to meals. With sweet, earthy flavors that combine with the toothsome bite of the barley, this salad makes a great side or a delicious lunch.

1 small butternut squash, peeled and diced

3 teaspoons, plus 2 tablespoons extra-virgin olive oil, divided

2 cups broccoli florets

1 cup pearl barley

2 cups baby kale

1 cup toasted chopped walnuts

½ red onion, sliced

2 tablespoons balsamic vinegar

2 garlic cloves, minced

½ teaspoon salt

¼ teaspoon freshly ground black pepper

1. Preheat the oven to 400°F. Line a baking sheet with parchment paper.

2. In a large bowl, toss the squash with 2 teaspoons of olive oil. Transfer to the prepared baking sheet and roast for 20 minutes.

3. While the squash is roasting, toss the broccoli in the same bowl with 1 teaspoon of olive oil. After 20 minutes, flip the squash and push it to one side of the baking sheet. Add the broccoli to the other side and continue to roast for 20 minutes more until tender.

4. While the veggies are roasting, in a medium pot, cover the barley with several inches of water. Bring to a boil, then reduce the heat, cover, and simmer for 30 minutes until tender. Drain and rinse.

5. Transfer the barley to a large bowl and toss with the cooked squash and broccoli, kale, walnuts, and onion.

6. In a small bowl, mix the remaining 2 tablespoons of olive oil, the balsamic vinegar, garlic, salt, and pepper. Toss the salad with the dressing and serve.

7. Store in the refrigerator for up to 3 days or freeze in individual servings for up to 6 months.

TIP: Butternut squash is one of the simplest winter squashes to prepare because its tough outer layer is easy to remove. Cut off one end of the squash so it stands upright on the cut end. Using a sharp knife or a vegetable peeler, start at the top of the squash and cut the skin off downward in strips, working around the squash, until it's peeled.

TIP: Add another protein source to complete this recipe. Grill or bake 2 or 3 ounces of your favorite lean protein at the same time the butternut squash is roasting.

Per Serving (about 1½ cups): Calories: 274; Protein: 6g; Total fat: 15g; Total carbohydrates: 32g; Fiber: 7g; Sugars: 3g; Sodium: 144mg; Iron: 2mg

Fattoush

Prep time: 10 minutes | **Cook time:** 10 minutes | Makes 8

Fattoush is a Middle Eastern bread salad that uses pita bread, veggies, and a zippy vinaigrette. It's a beautiful balance of acidity, hearty flavors, and fragrant herbs and spices that makes a truly satisfying salad to be enjoyed as a side item or as a meal.

4 whole-wheat pitas, chopped

2 tablespoons, plus ¼ cup extra-virgin olive oil

1 teaspoon lemon pepper, divided

1 head of butter lettuce, shredded

1 cucumber, chopped

1 pint cherry tomatoes, halved

1 bunch scallions, chopped

5 radishes, thinly sliced

3 tablespoons freshly squeezed lime juice

½ teaspoon sea salt

½ teaspoon ground cinnamon

¼ teaspoon ground allspice

1. Preheat the oven to 375°F. Line a baking sheet with parchment paper.

2. In a small bowl, mix the chopped pita with 2 tablespoons of olive oil and ½ teaspoon of lemon pepper. Mix well.

3. Spread in a single layer on the prepared baking sheet and bake in the oven until golden brown. Set aside to cool.

4. In a large bowl, combine the lettuce, cucumber, cherry tomatoes, scallions, and radishes.

5. Add the cooled pita bread and toss.

6. In a small bowl, whisk together the remaining ¼ cup of olive oil, ½ teaspoon of lemon pepper, the lime juice, salt, cinnamon, and allspice. Toss with the pita salad.

7. Store components separately. Store the pitas in a zip-top bag in a cupboard for up to 1 week. Store the salad tightly sealed in the refrigerator for up to 3 days. Store the dressing in a container in the refrigerator for up to 3 days. Toss all together to serve.

TIP: The traditional spice used with fattoush is sumac; if available, use that in place of the lemon pepper.

Per Serving (about 2 cups): Calories: 199; Protein: 4g; Total fat: 11g; Total carbohydrates: 23g; Fiber: 4g; Sugars: 3g; Sodium: 226mg; Iron: 2mg

Greek Salad

Prep time: 10 minutes | Makes 4

This Mediterranean Greek salad is bright, acidic, and aromatic with Greek-inspired herbs and spices along with plenty of fresh veggies. It makes a vibrant side salad, or when lean protein such as grilled chicken breast is added, it's the perfect main dish for a satisfying and delicious dinner.

1 head butter lettuce

1 cucumber, chopped

1 pint cherry tomatoes, halved

½ red onion, thinly sliced

½ cup black olives, chopped

¼ cup crumbled feta cheese

4 servings Greek Lemon Vinaigrette (page 126)

1. In a large bowl, combine the lettuce, cucumber, cherry tomatoes, onion, olives, and cheese. Mix.

2. Toss with the vinaigrette.

3. Store the dressing and salad separately, both in tightly sealed containers, in the refrigerator for up to 3 days. Toss before serving.

TIP: Traditionally, Kalamata olives are used in Greek salad; if available, replace the black olives with pitted Kalamatas for a more authentic experience.

Per Serving (about 2 cups): Calories: 224; Protein: 4g; Total fat: 18g; Total carbohydrates: 2g; Fiber: 1g; Sugars: 0g; Sodium: 94mg; Iron: 1mg

Chicken Chopped Salad

Prep time: 10 minutes, plus 6 hours to marinate | **Cook time:** 25 minutes | Makes 4

This chicken chopped salad is loaded with flavor, stores well, and is a convenient lunch or even a quick dinner. It's a delightful mix of textures and colors, with soft chicken and crunchy veggies along with a garlic and citrus tang from the creamy dressing. Up the crunch factor by adding grated carrots or even pre-packaged coleslaw mix.

2 boneless, skinless chicken breast halves

4 servings Greek Lemon Vinaigrette, divided (page 126)

1 head romaine lettuce

2 Roma tomatoes, chopped

1 red bell pepper, seeded, ribs removed, and chopped

1 zucchini, chopped

1 bunch scallions, chopped

¼ cup plain Greek yogurt

2 garlic cloves, minced

1 tablespoon red wine vinegar

1. In a zip-top bag, marinate the chicken breasts in two servings of the vinaigrette for 6 hours or overnight.

2. Preheat the oven to 400°F. Remove the chicken breasts from the vinaigrette and pat them dry. Place on a rimmed baking sheet and cook in the oven for 20 to 25 minutes, until the chicken reaches an internal temperature of 165°F. Let cool, then chop into cubes.

3. In a large bowl, combine the chicken, lettuce, tomatoes, bell pepper, zucchini, and scallions. Mix.

4. In a smaller bowl, whisk together the remaining two servings of lemon vinaigrette, the Greek yogurt, garlic, and red wine vinegar. Toss with the salad.

5. Store the dressing and salad separately, both in tightly sealed containers, in the refrigerator for up to 3 days. Toss before serving.

TIP: Double the vinaigrette recipe and make extra chicken while the oven is hot. Store the cooked unused chicken, chopped, in sealed zip-top bags in the freezer for up to 6 months and thaw for quick meals and salads.

Per Serving (about 2 cups): Calories: 132; Protein: 0g; Total fat: 14g; Total carbohydrates: 14g; Fiber: 5g; Sugars: 7g; Sodium: 316mg; Iron: 3mg

Oven-Roasted Eggplant Slices

Prep time: 5 minutes | **Cook time:** 30 minutes | Makes 4

Something magical happens when eggplant is roasted—it gets a soft, creamy consistency that picks up the flavors of whatever it is spiced with. These roasted eggplant slices make the perfect side item, or a great vegan meal by layering them with marinara for a lasagne-like main dish.

¼ cup extra-virgin olive oil

1 teaspoon garlic powder

1 teaspoon Italian seasoning

½ teaspoon sea salt

¼ teaspoon freshly ground black pepper

Pinch red pepper flakes (optional)

2 eggplants, cut into ½-inch-thick slices, unpeeled

1. Preheat the oven to 400°F. Line two rimmed baking sheets with parchment paper.

2. In a small bowl, whisk together the olive oil, garlic powder, Italian seasoning, salt, black pepper, and red pepper flakes.

3. Brush the mixture on both sides of the eggplant slices and place them in a single layer on the prepared baking sheets.

4. Bake in the oven until golden brown, 25 to 30 minutes.

5. Store in the refrigerator for up to 3 days.

TIP: Eggplant can be a little bitter because of the water it holds. To remove the bitter liquid, place the slices in a colander and sprinkle them liberally with salt. Put the colander in the sink and let it sit for about 20 minutes. With a paper towel, wipe or blot the salt away from the eggplant and continue the recipe as written. Omit the salt from the oil mixture.

Per Serving (½ eggplant): Calories: 190; Protein: 3g; Total fat: 14g; Total carbohydrates: 17g; Fiber: 8g; Sugars: 10g; Sodium: 152mg; Iron: 1mg

Apple-Ginger Slaw

Prep time: 10 minutes | Makes 4

This crisp slaw is sweet and tart with a subtle bite of ginger. It makes a delicious side salad with a refreshing flavor profile that's perfect to serve alongside rich foods to refresh the palate. Choose sweet-tart apples such as Cripps Pink, Braeburn, or Pink Lady apples for the perfect flavor balance.

4 apples, peeled, cored, and julienned

1 fennel bulb, cored and julienned

1 tablespoon freshly squeezed lemon juice

½ cup plain Greek yogurt

1 tablespoon grated fresh ginger

1 teaspoon apple cider vinegar

Pinch sea salt

1 teaspoon honey (optional)

1. In a large bowl, combine the apples and fennel. Toss with the lemon juice.

2. In a small bowl, whisk together the yogurt, ginger, vinegar, salt, and honey (if using).

3. Toss with the apples and fennel.

4. Store tightly sealed in the refrigerator for up to 3 days.

TIP: Save prep time by grating the apples on a box grater.

Per Serving (½ cup): Calories: 134; Protein: 2g; Total fat: 1g; Total carbohydrates: 31g; Fiber: 6g; Sugars: 23g; Sodium: 85mg; Iron: 1mg

Ponzu Grilled Avocado

Prep time: 5 minutes | **Cook time:** 5 minutes | Makes 4

This is a surprisingly delicious—and easy—side dish. The creamy, rich avocado balances beautifully with the tangy, salty ponzu sauce and the sesame seeds for a satisfying treat. This also works well as an appetizer, or serve it as a side for a simple soy-marinated fish or chicken dish.

2 avocadoes, peeled and pitted

4 servings Easy Ponzu Sauce (page 131)

1 tablespoon sesame seeds

1. Preheat a grill pan or grill on high.

2. Lightly brush the avocado halves on both sides with the ponzu sauce.

3. Place on the grill, cut-side down, and allow the grill to mark the avocado, 1 to 2 minutes. Turn the avocadoes over and mark the other side as well, another 1 to 2 minutes.

4. Put the avocadoes on plates and brush with the ponzu sauce. Fill the cavities with the remaining ponzu and sprinkle with the sesame seeds.

5. Store in zip-top bags in the refrigerator for up to 3 days.

TIP: To prep the avocadoes, halve each lengthwise and remove the pit. Then use a large spoon to scoop the avocadoes out of the peels.

Per Serving (½ avocado): Calories: 203; Protein: 4g; Total fat: 16g; Total carbohydrates: 15g; Fiber: 7g; Sugars: 5g; Sodium: 648mg; Iron: 1mg

Crispy Roasted Brussels Sprouts with Pine Nuts

Prep time: 10 minutes | **Cook time:** 30 minutes | Makes 4

Brussels sprouts have become the surprise star of restaurants and home cooking in recent years. But these aren't your parents' mushy Brussels sprouts. These are deeply flavored with delightfully crispy edges that are sure to convert even the strongest vegetable skeptic. Combined with a light balsamic glaze drizzle, they're sure to become a favorite.

1½ pounds Brussels sprouts, halved and trimmed

2 tablespoons extra-virgin olive oil

½ teaspoon sea salt

¼ teaspoon freshly ground black pepper

¼ cup balsamic vinegar

Juice and grated zest of ½ orange

1 tablespoon pure maple syrup

1 garlic clove, minced

¼ cup pine nuts

1. Preheat the oven to 400°F.

2. In a large bowl, toss the Brussels sprouts with the olive oil, salt, and pepper. Spread in a single layer on two rimmed baking sheets and roast in the oven until browned, 20 to 30 minutes.

3. While the Brussels sprouts are cooking, in a small saucepan, combine the balsamic vinegar, orange juice and zest, maple syrup, and garlic. Bring to a simmer over medium-high heat and simmer until thick and syrupy, about 10 minutes.

4. Put the roasted Brussels sprouts in a bowl. Toss with the pine nuts and the balsamic glaze.

5. Store leftovers in a zip-top bag in the refrigerator for up to 3 days.

TIP: To trim Brussels sprouts, cut off the bottom of the sprouts and halve vertically. Remove any browned leaves.

Per Serving (½ cup): Calories: 223; Protein: 7g; Total fat: 13g; Total carbohydrates: 24g; Fiber: 7g; Sugars: 10g; Sodium: 193mg; Iron: 3mg

Garlicky Green Beans

Prep time: 10 minutes | **Cook time:** 10 minutes | Makes 4

The trick to crisp-tender green beans lies in the blanching. It's easy to do—just stick them in boiling water for 5 minutes and then run them under cold water right away to stop the cooking. This leaves the beans bright green, slightly crisp, and ready to quickly cook with garlic for a delicious veggie side.

1 teaspoon sea salt

1 pound green beans, stemmed and halved

2 tablespoons extra-virgin olive oil

4 garlic cloves, minced

Grated zest of 1 lemon

1. Bring a large pot of water to a boil and add the sea salt.

2. Add the green beans and boil for 5 minutes.

3. Strain into a colander and immediately run under cold water to stop the cooking. Drain.

4. In a large skillet, heat the olive oil over medium-high heat until it shimmers. Add the green beans and cook, stirring, for 3 minutes.

5. Add the garlic and cook, stirring constantly, for 30 seconds.

6. Remove from the heat and stir in the lemon zest.

7. Store in the refrigerator for up to 3 days or in the freezer for up to 6 months.

TIP: When blanching green beans, use a large pot with enough water to cover the beans by at least an inch. Although water will seem salty with a whole teaspoon of salt in it, it will leave the beans only lightly salted.

Per Serving (½ cup): Calories: 99; Protein: 2g; Total fat: 7g; Total carbohydrates: 9g; Fiber: 3g; Sugars: 4g; Sodium: 298mg; Iron: 1mg

Chili Lime Coleslaw

Prep time: 10 minutes | Makes 4

This crisp coleslaw has a tart and spicy vinaigrette with just a hint of sweetness. It makes a great tangy side dish, but it's also delicious with grilled shrimp or chicken to make a yummy main. Chinese hot mustard powder can be found in either the spice section or the Asian section of the grocery store. If hot mustard is not a favorite, leave it out.

1 head cabbage, shredded

1 bunch scallions, thinly sliced

¼ cup chopped fresh cilantro

5 radishes, grated

1 carrot, grated

Juice of 2 limes

Grated zest of 1 lime

¼ cup extra-virgin olive oil

½ teaspoon Chinese hot mustard powder (optional)

½ teaspoon chipotle chili powder

1 teaspoon honey

1. In a large bowl, combine the cabbage, scallions, cilantro, radishes, and carrot. Mix.

2. In a small bowl, whisk together the lime juice and zest, olive oil, hot mustard powder (if using), chipotle chili powder, and honey. Toss with the slaw.

3. Store tightly sealed in the refrigerator for up to 3 days.

TIP: The fastest way to shred cabbage for coleslaw is to grate it on the large holes of a box grater.

Per Serving (½ cup): Calories: 201; Protein: 4g; Total fat: 14g; Total carbohydrates: 20g; Fiber: 7g; Sugars: 10g; Sodium: 68mg; Iron: 2mg

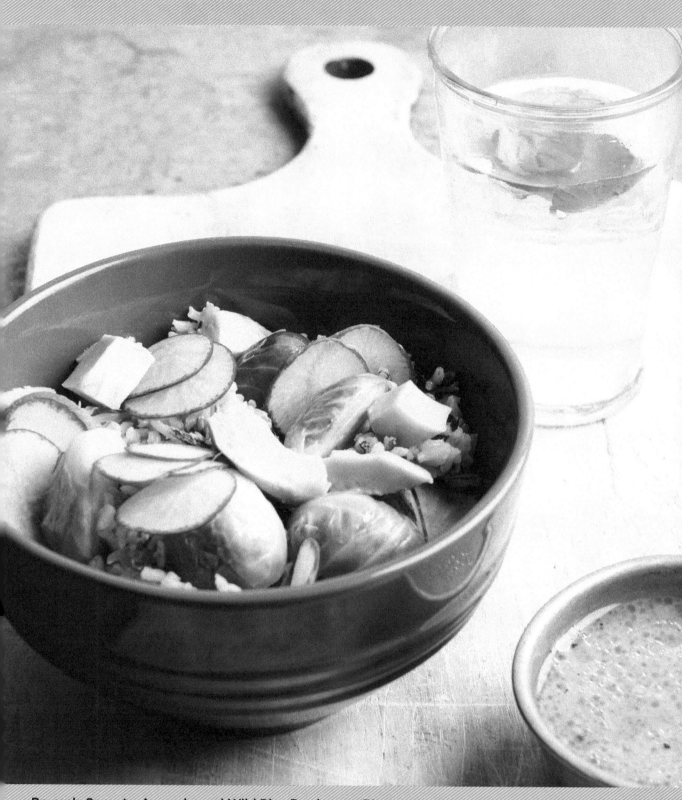

Brussels Sprouts, Avocado, and Wild Rice Bowl, page 72.

CHAPTER 6

Plant-Based Mains

Brussels Sprouts, Avocado, and Wild Rice Bowl

Prep time: 15 minutes | **Cook time:** 15 minutes | Makes 4

Wild rice has a nutty flavor that complements the toasty, caramelized Brussels sprouts. Meanwhile, avocado adds grassy notes and a creamy fattiness that serves as the ideal texture counterpoint, making these bowls a perfectly flavor-balanced meal.

2 cups sliced Brussels sprouts

2 teaspoons extra-virgin olive oil, plus 2 tablespoons

Juice of 1 lemon

1 teaspoon Dijon mustard

1 garlic clove, minced

½ teaspoon salt

¼ teaspoon freshly ground black pepper

1 cup cooked wild rice

1 cup sliced radishes

1 avocado, peeled, pitted, and sliced

1. Preheat the oven to 400°F. Line a baking sheet with parchment paper.

2. In a medium bowl, toss the Brussels sprouts with 2 teaspoons of olive oil and spread on the prepared baking sheet. Roast for 12 minutes, stirring once, until lightly browned.

3. In a small bowl, mix the remaining 2 tablespoons of olive oil, the lemon juice, mustard, garlic, salt, and pepper.

4. In a large bowl, toss the cooked wild rice, radishes, and roasted Brussels sprouts. Drizzle the dressing over the salad and toss.

5. Divide among four bowls and top with avocado slices.

6. Store these bowls without the avocadoes, and add the avocadoes just before serving. The rice and Brussels sprouts will keep in the refrigerator for up to 3 days or in the freezer for 6 months.

Per Serving (about 1 cup and ¼ avocado): Calories: 178; Protein: 2g; Total fat: 11g; Total carbohydrates: 18g; Fiber: 5g; Sugars: 2g; Sodium: 299mg; Iron: 1mg

Warm Soba and Tofu Bowl

Prep time: 20 minutes | **Cook time:** 10 minutes | Makes 4

There's a saying that we eat with our eyes first, and this salad supports that notion. The brightly colored veggies are enticing and satisfying. The dish is a flavor and texture explosion that's so balanced and beautiful, the meat won't be missed.

8 ounces soba noodles

3 tablespoons orange juice

2 tablespoons low-sodium yellow mustard

1 tablespoon lemon juice

1 tablespoon pure maple syrup

1 teaspoon dried thyme

⅛ teaspoon black pepper

1 tablespoon sesame oil

8 ounces firm tofu, drained and cut into 1-inch pieces

3 cups chopped red cabbage

1 red bell pepper, seeded, ribs removed, and chopped

1 carrot, grated

3 scallions, chopped

4 cups mixed salad greens

1. Bring a large pot of water to a boil. Add the soba noodles and cook according to the package directions. Drain, rinse with warm water, drain again, and put into a serving bowl.

2. Meanwhile, in a small bowl, combine the orange juice, mustard, lemon juice, maple syrup, thyme, and black pepper and mix well.

3. Heat a large nonstick skillet over medium heat. Add the sesame oil.

4. Add the tofu cubes and cook for 2 minutes, stirring occasionally.

5. Add the cabbage, bell pepper, and carrot. Cook and stir for 3 to 4 minutes longer. Add the orange juice mixture and bring to a simmer.

6. Put the tofu and vegetable mixture and scallions in the serving bowl with the soba noodles and toss. Serve over the salad greens.

7. Store this with the salad greens separately in the refrigerator for up to 3 days.

TIP: Watch out for the sodium content in soba noodles; many can provide 25 percent of the daily sodium consumption in just one 2-ounce serving!

Per Serving (1 bowl): Calories: 343; Protein: 17g; Total fat: 8g; Total carbohydrates: 59g; Fiber: 4g; Sugars: 10g; Sodium: 574mg; Iron: 4mg

Whole-Wheat Pasta Puttanesca

Prep time: 10 minutes | **Cook time:** 15 minutes | Makes 4

Puttanesca is a traditional Italian tomato-based pasta sauce. The addition of olives and capers adds a punch of flavor and texture that makes this an especially satisfying pasta sauce. Don't skip the fragrant garnish (called gremolata) at the end; it adds a ton of flavor and aromatics.

2 tablespoons extra-virgin olive oil

½ yellow onion, finely chopped

6 garlic cloves, minced, divided

1 (28-ounce) can diced tomatoes

⅓ cup chopped black olives

2 tablespoons capers, drained

2 tablespoons Italian seasoning

8 ounces whole-wheat spaghetti (or any whole-wheat pasta), cooked according to the package directions and drained

¼ cup chopped fresh parsley

Grated zest of 1 lemon

1. In a large rimmed skillet, heat the olive oil over medium-high until it shimmers.

2. Add the onion and cook until soft, about 3 minutes.

3. Add 5 of the minced garlic cloves and cook, stirring constantly, for 30 seconds.

4. Add the tomatoes with their juices, olives, capers, and Italian seasoning. Bring to a simmer, stirring occasionally, and reduce the heat to medium-low.

5. Simmer for 10 minutes, stirring occasionally.

6. Spoon over the cooked spaghetti.

7. In a small bowl, mix together the parsley, lemon zest, and remaining minced garlic clove. Sprinkle over the pasta and sauce as a garnish.

8. Store pasta and sauce mixed together in individual portions in the refrigerator for up to 5 days or in the freezer for up to 6 months. Make the garnish fresh.

TIP: You can use zucchini noodles instead of whole-wheat ones. Use a peeler to peel the zucchini into ribbons and then cut them into noodle strips using a sharp knife. Add them to the sauce in the last 5 minutes of simmering.

Per Serving (1 cup pasta, ½ cup sauce): Calories: 319; Protein: 11g; Total fat: 9g; Total carbohydrates: 54g; Fiber: 9g; Sugars: 6g; Sodium: 211mg; Iron: 4mg

Quinoa and Veggie Stuffed Zucchini

Prep time: 10 minutes | **Cook time:** 20 minutes | Makes 4

Quinoa has a nutty flavor and a hearty bite that make these Tex-Mex–inspired zucchini boats satisfying. Precook the quinoa and freeze it in 1-cup servings in zip-top bags; it's a great way to have prepped food ready to go.

4 medium zucchini, halved lengthwise

2 tablespoons extra-virgin olive oil

1 onion, finely chopped

1 green bell pepper, seeded, ribs removed, and chopped

3 garlic cloves, minced

1 (14-ounce) can black beans, drained

1 (14-ounce) can diced tomatoes, drained

1 cup cooked quinoa

1 teaspoon chipotle chili powder

½ teaspoon sea salt

1. Preheat the oven to 425°F. Partially hollow out the zucchini halves using a teaspoon. Chop the removed zucchini section and set aside. Place the hollowed halves, cut-side up, on a rimmed baking sheet.

2. In a large skillet, heat the olive oil over medium-high until it shimmers.

3. Add the chopped zucchini, onion, and bell pepper and cook until soft, 3 to 5 minutes. Add the garlic and cook, stirring constantly, for 30 seconds.

4. Add the black beans, diced tomatoes, quinoa, chili powder, and salt. Cook, stirring, until everything is warmed through, about 5 minutes.

5. Spoon the mixture into the zucchini boats. Bake in the oven until the zucchini is soft, 15 to 20 minutes.

6. Store, tightly wrapped, in the refrigerator for up to 5 days or in the freezer for up to 6 months.

TIP: For tastier quinoa, rinse it before cooking. Rinse in a mesh colander under cool running water, rubbing the grains between your fingers. Fully drain before cooking.

Per Serving (2 boats): Calories: 272; Protein: 12g; Total fat: 9g; Total carbohydrates: 40g; Fiber: 12g; Sugars: 10g; Sodium: 197mg; Iron: 4mg

Butternut Squash Soup with Pepitas

Prep time: 10 minutes | **Cook time:** 25 minutes | Makes 6

Earthy and sweet, butternut squash soup works well with fragrant herbs and spices to make a deeply warming, heartily satisfying soup. This is a great recipe to double batch because it freezes so well and can be a quick, warm, and flavorful meal.

2 tablespoons extra-virgin olive oil

1 onion, minced

1 butternut squash, peeled and chopped into ½-inch cubes

2 garlic cloves

4 cups low-sodium vegetable broth

1 teaspoon grated ginger

1 teaspoon ground sage

½ teaspoon sea salt

¼ teaspoon freshly ground black pepper

¼ cup pepitas

1. In a large pot, heat the olive oil over medium-high until it shimmers.

2. Add the onion and cook until it begins to soften, about 3 minutes. Add the squash and cook until it begins to soften, about 7 minutes more. Add the garlic and cook, stirring constantly, for 30 seconds.

3. Add the vegetable broth, ginger, sage, salt, and pepper. Bring to a boil and reduce the heat to medium-low.

4. Cover and simmer until the squash is soft, 15 to 20 minutes.

5. Very carefully transfer to a blender. Blend to puree.

6. Serve sprinkled with pepitas.

7. Store in individual servings in the refrigerator for up to 5 days or in the freezer for up to 6 months.

TIP: When pureeing the soup, be careful not to get burned. Pour the hot soup into the blender and put the lid on. Fold a towel and place it over the top of the blender, then puree for 20 seconds. Be sure to vent the steam by opening the lid. Cover again, and puree for 30 seconds, venting again. Put the lid back on and puree until smooth.

Per Serving (about 1 cup of soup): Calories: 140; Protein: 3g; Total fat: 7g; Total carbohydrates: 19g; Fiber: 4g; Sugars: 4g; Sodium: 104mg; Iron: 1mg

Southwestern Black Bean Chili

Prep time: 10 minutes | **Cook time:** 20 minutes | Makes 6

Everyone needs a hearty chili recipe in their back pocket. This version makes the most of Tex-Mex flavors and the hearty bite of black beans as a spicy and satisfying main dish. If you prefer your chili on the spicier side, add some cayenne as it simmers.

2 tablespoons extra-virgin olive oil

1 onion, chopped

1 green bell pepper, seeded, ribs removed, and chopped

4 garlic cloves

2 (14-ounce) cans black beans, drained

1 (28-ounce) can diced tomatoes

2 tablespoons chili powder

1 teaspoon ground cumin

½ teaspoon dried oregano

½ teaspoon sea salt

1. In a large pot, heat the olive oil over medium-high heat until it shimmers.

2. Add the onion and bell pepper and cook until they begin to soften, about 3 minutes.

3. Add the garlic and cook, stirring constantly, for 30 seconds.

4. Add the black beans, tomatoes with their juices, chili powder, cumin, oregano, and salt. Bring to a simmer.

5. Reduce the heat to medium-low and simmer, stirring occasionally, for 10 minutes.

6. Store in individual servings in the refrigerator for up to 5 days or in the freezer for up to 6 months.

TIP: For a smokier chili, add either 1 teaspoon of smoked paprika or ½ teaspoon of chipotle chili powder along with the other spices in step 4.

Per Serving (about 1 cup of soup): Calories: 198; Protein: 10g; Total fat: 6g; Total carbohydrates: 30g; Fiber: 12g; Sugars: 5g; Sodium: 190mg; Iron: 3mg

Minestrone Soup

Prep time: 15 minutes | **Cook time:** 30 minutes | Makes 6

Minestrone is a hearty Italian vegetable soup aromatic with herbs, garlic, and spices. Feel free to add any fresh veggies to this basic mix. Some excellent add-ins include summer squash, chopped fennel bulb, and peas.

2 tablespoons extra-virgin olive oil

1 onion, chopped

1 red bell pepper, seeded, ribs removed, and chopped

2 carrots, chopped

1 cup green beans, stemmed and halved

4 garlic cloves

1 (14-ounce) can diced tomatoes

1 (14-ounce) can kidney beans, drained

4 cups low-sodium vegetable broth

1 tablespoon dried Italian seasoning

½ teaspoon sea salt

1 cup whole-wheat elbow macaroni

1. In a large pot, heat the olive oil over medium-high heat until it shimmers.

2. Add the onion, bell pepper, carrots, and green beans and cook, stirring occasionally, until the veggies begin to soften, about 5 minutes.

3. Add the garlic and cook, stirring constantly, for 30 seconds.

4. Add the tomatoes with their juices, kidney beans, vegetable broth, Italian seasoning, and salt. Bring to a boil, stirring occasionally.

5. Add the elbow macaroni and bring the mixture back to a boil. Reduce the heat to medium-low and simmer until the macaroni is tender, about 10 minutes.

6. Store in individual servings in the refrigerator for up to 5 days or in the freezer for up to 6 months.

TIP: Want a bit of spice? Add a few pinches of red pepper flakes along with the other seasonings in step 4.

Per Serving (about 2 cups of soup): Calories: 197; Protein: 8g; Total fat: 5g; Total carbohydrates: 32g; Fiber: 7g; Sugars: 5g; Sodium: 192mg; Iron: 2mg

Lebanese-Inspired Chickpea Stew

Prep time: 15 minutes | **Cook time:** 30 minutes | Makes 4

This aromatic stew is a perfect fall or winter warmer. Hearty chickpeas soak up the flavors of the Lebanese-inspired spices, creating a tender stew that tastes as good as it smells. With such a powerful flavor profile, it's certain to become a favorite.

2 tablespoons extra-virgin olive oil

1 onion, chopped

1 red bell pepper, seeded, ribs removed, and chopped

4 garlic cloves, minced

1 teaspoon ground cumin

1 teaspoon dried thyme

1 teaspoon ground paprika

2 cups low-sodium vegetable broth

2 (14-ounce) cans chickpeas, drained

½ teaspoon salt

Grated zest of 1 lemon

¼ cup chopped fresh parsley

1. In a large pot, heat the olive oil over medium-high heat until it shimmers.

2. Add the onion and bell pepper and cook until the veggies begin to soften, 3 to 5 minutes.

3. Add the garlic, cumin, thyme, and paprika and cook, stirring constantly, for 30 seconds.

4. Add the vegetable broth, chickpeas, and salt. Bring to a simmer and reduce the heat to medium low. Simmer, stirring occasionally, for 10 minutes.

5. Stir in the lemon zest and parsley just before serving.

6. Store in individual servings in the refrigerator for up to 5 days or in the freezer for up to 6 months.

TIP: Make this more authentic by adding za'atar spice. Replace the thyme with 2 teaspoons of za'atar.

Per Serving (about 1 cup stew): Calories: 291; Protein: 12g; Total fat: 10g; Total carbohydrates: 40g; Fiber: 11g; Sugars: 8g; Sodium: 160mg; Iron: 5mg

Lentil Curry

Prep time: 10 minutes | **Cook time:** 30 minutes | Makes 4

Sweet potatoes and lentils are the perfect backdrop for the curry spices used in this quick stew. The curry and garlic make the stew fragrant, while the lentils and sweet potatoes add an earthy sweetness that makes this dish so deeply satisfying.

2 tablespoons extra-virgin olive oil

1 onion, chopped

4 garlic cloves, minced

1 teaspoon grated ginger

3 cups low-sodium vegetable broth

2 (14-ounce) cans lentils, drained

1 (14-ounce) can diced tomatoes, drained

2 sweet potatoes, cut into ½-inch cubes

1 tablespoon curry powder

½ teaspoon sea salt

1. In a large pot, heat the olive oil over medium-high heat until it shimmers.

2. Add the onion and cook until it softens, about 3 minutes.

3. Add the garlic and ginger and cook, stirring constantly, for 30 seconds.

4. Add the vegetable broth, lentils, tomatoes, sweet potatoes, curry powder, and salt. Bring to a boil. Reduce the heat to medium-low and cover.

5. Simmer until the potatoes are soft, about 20 minutes.

6. Store in individual servings in the refrigerator for up to 5 days or in the freezer for up to 6 months.

TIP: Leave the sweet potatoes unpeeled for this recipe; doing so adds fiber, which makes the dish even more filling and satisfying.

Per Serving (about 1½ cups): Calories: 325; Protein: 16g; Total fat: 8g; Total carbohydrates: 51g; Fiber: 17g; Sugars: 9g; Sodium: 197mg; Iron: 6mg

Whole-Wheat Veggie Pasta with Basil Pesto

Prep time: 10 minutes | **Cook time:** 10 minutes | Makes 4

Pesto is a super easy sauce that can be made in about 5 minutes. For a super quick meal, mix up a batch of pesto and toss it with fresh, hot pasta. Or spruce it up with additional veggies for a colorful, filling, tasty meal.

2 tablespoons extra-virgin olive oil

1 onion, chopped

2 carrots, chopped

2 cups broccoli florets or broccolini

1 red bell pepper, seeded, ribs removed, and chopped

½ teaspoon sea salt

Pinch red pepper flakes

3 garlic cloves, minced

8 ounces whole-wheat spaghetti, cooked according to the package directions and drained

3½ cups Basil Pesto (page 124)

1. In a large nonstick skillet, heat the olive oil over medium-high heat until it shimmers.

2. Add the onion, carrots, broccoli, bell pepper, salt, and red pepper flakes and cook, stirring occasionally, until the veggies are crisp-tender, 7 to 10 minutes.

3. Add the garlic and cook, stirring constantly, for 30 seconds.

4. In a large bowl, toss the veggies with the pasta and the pesto until well mixed.

5. Store in individual servings in the refrigerator for up to 5 days or in the freezer for up to 6 months.

TIP: Adjust the heat level up or down by omitting red pepper flakes or adding them to taste. They are quite spicy, so add just a pinch at a time.

Per Serving (about 1½ cups): Calories: 487; Protein: 11g; Total fat: 37g; Total carbohydrates: 29g; Fiber: 6g; Sugars: 5g; Sodium: 567mg; Iron: 1mg

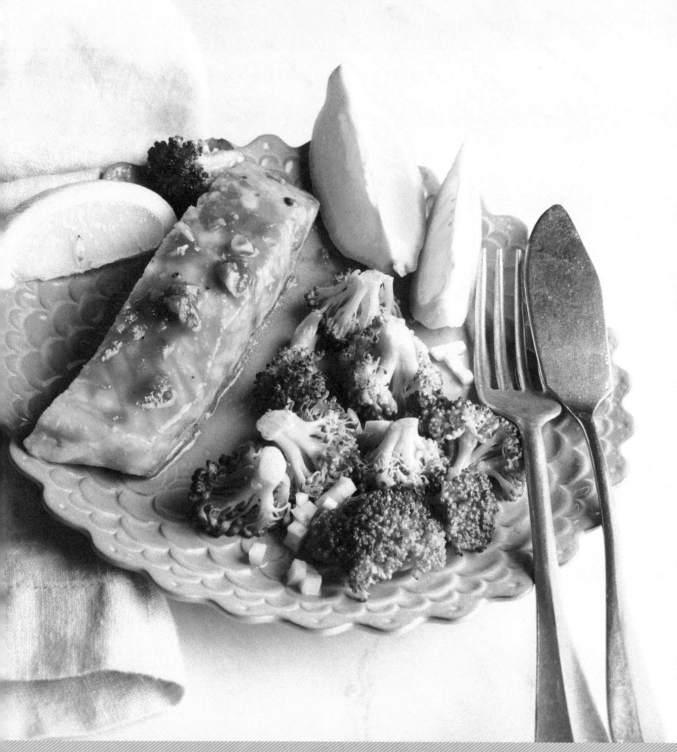

Ginger-Glazed Salmon with Broccoli, page 84.

CHAPTER 7

Fish and Seafood

Ginger-Glazed Salmon with Broccoli

Prep time: 10 minutes | **Cook time:** 15 minutes | Makes 4

Salmon is full of omega-3 fatty acids, and ginger is a powerful anti-inflammatory spice. So not only is this dish delicious, it's nutritious.

Nonstick cooking spray

1 tablespoon low-sodium tamari or gluten-free soy sauce

Juice of 1 lemon

1 tablespoon honey

1 (1-inch) piece fresh ginger, grated

1 garlic clove, minced

1 pound salmon fillet

¼ teaspoon salt, divided

⅛ teaspoon freshly ground black pepper

2 broccoli heads, cut into florets

1 tablespoon extra-virgin olive oil

1. Preheat the oven to 400°F. Spray a baking sheet with nonstick cooking spray.

2. In a small bowl, mix the tamari, lemon juice, honey, ginger, and garlic. Set aside.

3. Place the salmon, skin-side down, on the prepared baking sheet. Season with ⅛ teaspoon of salt and the pepper.

4. In a large mixing bowl, toss the broccoli and olive oil. Season with the remaining ⅛ teaspoon of salt. Arrange in a single layer on the baking sheet next to the salmon. Bake for 15 to 20 minutes, until the salmon flakes easily with a fork and the broccoli is fork-tender.

5. In a small pan over medium heat, bring the tamari-ginger mixture to a simmer and cook for 1 to 2 minutes until it just begins to thicken.

6. Drizzle the sauce over the salmon and serve.

7. Store in the refrigerator for up to 3 days. This does not freeze well.

Per Serving (4 ounces salmon and ½ cup broccoli): Calories: 238; Protein: 25g; Total fat: 11g; Total carbohydrates: 11g; Fiber: 2g; Sugars: 6g; Sodium: 334mg; Iron: 3mg

Shrimp and Pineapple Lettuce Wraps

Prep time: 15 minutes | **Cook time:** 12 minutes | Makes 4

Subtly sweet shrimp pairs beautifully with the bright, tropical flavors of pineapple. With light heat, sweetness, and plenty of acid, these pineapple shrimp wraps make a quick and delightful seafood supper with a little bit of tropical flare.

2 teaspoons extra-virgin olive oil

2 jalapeño peppers, seeded and minced

6 scallions, chopped

2 yellow bell peppers, seeded, ribs removed, and chopped

8 ounces small shrimp, peeled and deveined

2 cups canned pineapple chunks, drained, reserving juice

2 tablespoons freshly squeezed lime juice

1 avocado, peeled, pitted, and cubed

1 large carrot, coarsely grated

8 romaine or Boston lettuce leaves, rinsed and patted dry

1. In a medium saucepan, heat the olive oil over medium heat.

2. Add the jalapeño peppers and scallions and cook for 2 minutes, stirring constantly.

3. Add the bell peppers and cook for 2 minutes.

4. Add the shrimp and cook for 1 minute, stirring constantly.

5. Add the pineapple, 2 tablespoons of reserved pineapple juice, and the lime juice and bring to a simmer. Simmer for 1 minute longer or until the shrimp curl and turn pink. Let the mixture cool for 5 minutes.

6. Serve the shrimp mixture with the avocado and carrot, wrapped in the lettuce leaves.

7. Store in the refrigerator for up to 3 days, with the shrimp mixture stored separately from the lettuce.

TIP: If needed, make the shrimp mixture up to 2 hours ahead of time; any longer, and the shrimp may become mushy. Store the mixture covered in the refrigerator. Warm the filling or serve it cold or at room temperature.

Per Serving (about 2 wraps): Calories: 230; Protein: 11g; Total fat: 11g; Total carbohydrates: 27g; Fiber: 7g; Sugars: 11g; Sodium: 347mg; Iron: 2mg

Lemony Mussels and Fennel

Prep time: 15 minutes | **Cook time:** 10 minutes | Makes 4

When heading to the seashore isn't possible, at least eat like the sand is between your toes. Sweet, briny mussels blend with the subtle anise flavor of fennel and the bright acidity of lemon to create a fast and easy, restaurant-quality weeknight meal.

2 tablespoons extra-virgin olive oil

1 red onion, minced

1 fennel bulb, cored finely, chopped, plus 2 tablespoons chopped fennel fronds

3 garlic cloves, minced

2 cups low-sodium vegetable broth

Juice and grated zest of 1 lemon

1 pound mussels in shells, rinsed

Pinch red pepper flakes

½ teaspoon sea salt

¼ teaspoon freshly ground black pepper

2 cups cooked brown rice

1. In a large pot, heat the olive oil over medium heat until it shimmers.

2. Add the onion and fennel and cook, stirring occasionally, until the veggies are soft, 3 to 5 minutes.

3. Add the garlic and cook, stirring constantly, for 30 seconds.

4. Add the vegetable broth, lemon juice and zest, mussels, red pepper flakes, salt, and black pepper. Bring to a boil.

5. Reduce the heat to medium-high and cover. Cook until the mussels open, about 5 minutes.

6. Spoon the sauce over the rice and serve the mussels on the side.

7. These mussels are best eaten fresh, but if needed, they can be stored in the refrigerator for up to 3 days. Don't freeze.

TIP: Replace the mussels with 1 pound of steamer clams. They take about the same amount of time to cook.

Per Serving (about ¼ pound mussels and ½ cup rice): Calories: 234; Protein: 8g; Total fat: 9g; Total carbohydrates: 32g; Fiber: 4g; Sugars: 4g; Sodium: 284mg; Iron: 2mg

Baked Cod Packets with Summer Squash

Prep time: 10 minutes | **Cook time:** 18 minutes | Makes 4

Baking cod in parchment paper or foil packets results in tender, moist fish packed with flavor. It's the perfect way to cook all kinds of fish—not just cod. This recipe calls for summer squash, but you can try sliced bell peppers, sliced fennel, carrots, or broccolini.

3 medium zucchini or another summer squash, thinly sliced

2 tablespoons extra-virgin olive oil, plus 2 teaspoons

4 (4-ounce) cod fillets, pin bones removed

1 teaspoon dried dill

½ teaspoon sea salt

¼ teaspoon freshly ground black pepper

Grated zest of 1 lemon

4 tablespoons freshly squeezed lemon juice

1. Preheat the oven to 400°F.

2. In a large bowl, toss the zucchini with 2 tablespoons of olive oil. Arrange in mounds on four 12 x 12-inch pieces of foil.

3. Place the cod on top of the zucchini and brush with the remaining 2 teaspoons of olive oil. Season with the dill, salt, pepper, and lemon zest.

4. Carefully fold the foil into packets, leaving the tops unsealed. Place the packets on a rimmed baking sheet.

5. Add 1 tablespoon of lemon juice to each packet and then seal the packet closed.

6. Bake in the oven until the fish is opaque and flaky, 15 to 18 minutes.

7. Store the fish in their foil packets in the refrigerator for up to 3 days. Don't freeze.

TIP: For a Southwestern take, replace the dill with chopped fresh cilantro, and the lemon zest and juice with lime zest and juice. Sprinkle each fillet with about ¼ teaspoon of chili powder when adding the salt and pepper in step 3.

Per Serving (1 packet): Calories: 186; Protein: 19g; Total fat: 10g; Total carbohydrates: 6g; Fiber: 2g; Sugars: 4g; Sodium: 487mg; Iron: 1mg

Weeknight Cioppino

Prep time: 10 minutes | **Cook time:** 25 minutes | Makes 4

This hearty fish stew has a rich, fragrant tomato-based broth flavored with fish, shrimp, and Italian seasoning. And although it sounds complicated, this dish comes together quickly, and the kitchen smells amazing while it cooks. It's enough to make any week-night seem like a special occasion.

2 tablespoons extra-virgin olive oil

1 onion, chopped

1 red bell pepper, seeded, ribs removed, and chopped

5 garlic cloves, minced

2 cups low-sodium vegetable broth

1 (14-ounce) can tomato sauce

1 tablespoon Italian seasoning

½ teaspoon sea salt

8 ounces skinless cod fillets, skin and bones removed and cut into ½-inch pieces

8 ounces medium shrimp, tails removed and deveined

Pinch red pepper flakes

¼ cup chopped fresh parsley

1. In a large pot, heat the olive oil over medium-high heat until it shimmers.

2. Add the onion and bell pepper and cook, stirring occasionally, until the veggies begin to soften, 3 to 5 minutes.

3. Add the garlic and cook, stirring constantly, for 30 seconds.

4. Add the vegetable broth, tomato sauce, Italian seasoning, and salt. Bring to a boil, stirring occasionally.

5. Add the cod, shrimp, and red pepper flakes. Return to a boil, stirring occasionally.

6. Reduce the heat to medium-low and simmer until the fish is opaque and the shrimp is pink, 5 to 7 minutes. Remove from the heat and stir in the parsley.

7. Store in individual servings in the refrigerator for up to 3 days or in the freezer for up to 6 months.

TIP: Try salmon (skin removed), clams, or even trout in place of the shrimp or cod. Just don't exceed 1 pound total of seafood.

Per Serving (about 1½ cups): Calories: 190; Protein: 22g; Total fat: 8g; Total carbohydrates: 9g; Fiber: 3g; Sugars: 5g; Sodium: 457mg; Iron: 1mg

Fast Fish Tacos

Prep time: 10 minutes | **Cook time:** 15 minutes | Makes 4

Any white fish works well for this recipe, so try cod, halibut, or whatever is locally available. Lettuce wraps replace corn tortillas, but the guacamole and mango salsa add tons of flavor so that the taco shells won't be missed. Butter lettuce works best here, as it is the most flexible and wraps well around the fish.

Juice and grated zest of
  1 lime

2 tablespoons
  extra-virgin olive oil,
  divided

1 tablespoon chili
  powder

½ teaspoon cumin

½ teaspoon sea salt

1 pound white-fleshed
  fish, pin bones and skin
  removed and cut into
  ½-inch pieces

8 butter lettuce leaves

4 servings Mango Salsa
  (page 127)

4 servings Guacamole
  (page 128)

1. In a medium bowl, whisk together the lime juice and zest, 1 tablespoon of olive oil, the chili powder, cumin, and salt. Add the fish and stir to coat. Allow to sit for 10 minutes.

2. In a large nonstick skillet, heat the remaining 1 tablespoon of olive oil over medium-high heat until it shimmers.

3. Remove the fish from the marinade and pat dry with paper towels. Add to the hot pan and cook, stirring occasionally, until the fish is opaque, 5 to 7 minutes.

4. Spoon the fish onto the butter lettuce and top with the mango salsa and guacamole.

5. Store the fish separately from the lettuce, salsa, and guacamole in the refrigerator for up to 3 days. Assemble just before eating.

TIP: Try making the guacamole and salsa ahead of time so baking the fish is all that's needed on the nights when there is a time crunch.

Per Serving (about 2 tacos): Calories: 297; Protein: 24g; Total fat: 16g; Total carbohydrates: 18g; Fiber: 6g; Sugars: 8g; Sodium: 513mg; Iron: 1mg

Oven-Baked Orange Salmon and Peppers

Prep time: 10 minutes | **Cook time:** 20 minutes | Makes 4

The pink flesh of the salmon and the colorful bell peppers are as pleasing to look at as they are to eat. Best of all, it can be made on a sheet pan, so cleanup is easy. It's a nutritious and fast meal that's perfect for busy weeknights.

3 bell peppers (1 red, 1 orange, 1 yellow), seeded, ribs removed, and thinly sliced

4 (4-ounce) salmon fillets

Juice of 1 orange and grated zest of ½ orange

1 teaspoon dried dill

1 teaspoon garlic powder

½ teaspoon sea salt

¼ teaspoon freshly ground black pepper

1. Preheat the oven to 400°F. Line a rimmed baking sheet with parchment paper.

2. Arrange the bell pepper pieces and salmon on the baking sheet.

3. In a small bowl, whisk together the orange juice and zest, dill, garlic powder, salt, and black pepper.

4. Drizzle the orange mixture over the salmon and peppers.

5. Bake in the oven until the salmon is pink and opaque and the peppers are crisp-tender, about 20 minutes.

6. Store the fish and peppers separately in the refrigerator for up to 3 days.

TIP: If allergic to fish but not shellfish, this works super well with shrimp, too. Reduce the cooking time by about 5 minutes.

Per Serving (1 fillet and about ¼ cup of peppers): Calories: 201; Protein: 24g; Total fat: 8g; Total carbohydrates: 8g; Fiber: 2g; Sugars: 6g; Sodium: 199mg; Iron: 1mg

Shrimp Fried Cauliflower Rice

Prep time: 10 minutes | **Cook time:** 18 minutes | Makes 4

Shrimp fried cauliflower rice is one of life's simple pleasures. Fragrant with Asian-inspired spices, it makes a delicious main course. Replacing the rice with riced cauliflower adds flavor and is much lower in calories and carbs than rice, making it a great rice substitute for those who are looking to drop a few pounds.

2 tablespoons extra-virgin olive oil

1 bunch scallions, chopped

1 carrot, chopped

1 pound medium shrimp, peeled, deveined, and tails removed

1 tablespoon grated ginger

3 garlic cloves, minced

1 egg, beaten

4 servings Cauliflower Rice (page 132)

1 tablespoon low-sodium soy sauce

1. In a large, nonstick skillet, heat the olive oil over medium-high heat until it shimmers.

2. Add the scallions and carrot and cook, stirring occasionally, until the veggies begin to brown, 5 to 7 minutes.

3. Add the shrimp and ginger and cook, stirring, until the shrimp is opaque, 3 to 5 minutes more.

4. Add the garlic and cook, stirring constantly, for 30 seconds.

5. Add the egg and cook, stirring, until the egg sets, about 2 minutes.

6. Add the cauliflower rice and soy sauce. Cook, stirring occasionally, until the rice is tender, about 5 minutes more.

7. Store in the refrigerator for up to 3 days or the freezer for up to 6 months.

TIP: Feel free to add more veggies to this recipe, cooking them with the scallions and the carrot. Tender peas are a great addition, as are green beans and broccoli florets.

Per Serving (about 2 cups): Calories: 289; Protein: 28g; Total fat: 16g; Total carbohydrates: 11g; Fiber: 4g; Sugars: 4g; Sodium: 485mg; Iron: 2mg

White Fish and Mushroom Mojo

Prep time: 10 minutes | **Cook time:** 30 minutes | Makes 4

This Southwestern-flavored fish dish uses any white-fleshed fish, so feel free to pick a favorite. Because the garlic is slowly cooked in oil over low heat, both the garlic and oil develop sweet flavors similar to roasted garlic. This flavors the fish and other ingredients for a deeply aromatic and satisfying meal.

¼ cup extra-virgin olive oil

8 garlic cloves, sliced

1 onion, chopped

8 ounces button mushrooms, quartered

1 pound white-fleshed fish fillets, bones and skin removed and cut into ½-inch pieces

1 teaspoon chili powder

½ teaspoon sea salt

Juice of 1 lime

¼ cup chopped fresh cilantro

2 cups cooked brown rice

1. In a small pot, heat the olive oil and garlic over low heat. Bring to barely a simmer (just one or two bubbles rising). Allow to simmer for 15 minutes, until the garlic is soft and golden.

2. Remove from the heat and cool slightly. Mash the garlic into the olive oil with a fork.

3. Take 2 tablespoons of the garlic oil and put it in a nonstick skillet over medium-high heat.

4. Add the onion and mushrooms. Cook, stirring occasionally, until the mushrooms begin to brown, 5 to 7 minutes.

5. Add the fish, chili powder, salt, lime juice, and remaining 2 tablespoons of garlic oil. Cook, stirring, until the fish is opaque, about 5 minutes more.

6. Remove from the heat and stir in the cilantro. Spoon over the rice.

7. Store in the refrigerator for up to 3 days.

TIP: If available, this recipe can be completed in a slow cooker on low for 2 to 3 hours.

Per Serving (4 ounces fish and ½ cup rice): Calories: 349; Protein: 24g; Total fat: 15g; Total carbohydrates: 30g; Fiber: 3g; Sugars: 3g; Sodium: 317mg; Iron: 1mg

Scampi and Garlic Zoodles

Prep time: 10 minutes | **Cook time:** 15 minutes | Makes 4

Scampi is another delightful Italian dish that's naturally light but full of flavor. Use any size shrimp for this recipe, just adjust the cooking times accordingly. For something a little heartier, replace the zoodles with cooked whole-wheat spaghetti.

3 tablespoons extra-virgin olive oil, divided

3 medium zucchini, peeled lengthwise into long ribbons, skin left on

½ red onion, minced

6 garlic cloves, minced

1 pound shrimp, peeled, deveined, and tails removed

Juice and grated zest of 1 lemon

1 cup low-sodium vegetable broth

Pinch red pepper flakes

½ teaspoon sea salt

¼ teaspoon freshly ground black pepper

¼ cup chopped fresh Italian parsley

1. In a large nonstick skillet, heat 2 tablespoons of olive oil over medium-high heat. Add the zucchini and cook, stirring occasionally, until tender, about 5 minutes. Remove from the pan and set aside.

2. Add the remaining 1 tablespoon of olive oil to the pan and heat until it shimmers. Add the onion and cook, stirring occasionally, until soft, about 3 minutes.

3. Add the garlic and cook, stirring constantly, for 30 seconds.

4. Add the shrimp, lemon juice and zest, vegetable broth, red pepper flakes, salt, and black pepper. Cook, stirring occasionally, until the shrimp is pink and opaque, 5 to 7 minutes.

5. Return the zucchini to the pan. Cook for a minute or two more to reheat the zucchini.

6. Remove from the heat and stir in the parsley.

7. Store in the refrigerator for up to 3 days.

TIP: This recipe uses zucchini ribbons, so the strips will be quite wide. If narrower strips are preferred, stack them and use a sharp knife to halve them lengthwise for a shape more like fettuccine.

Per Serving (4 ounces fish, ½ cup rice): Calories: 227; Protein: 25g; Total fat: 11g; Total carbohydrates: 8g; Fiber: 2g; Sugars: 5g; Sodium: 296mg; Iron: 2mg

Trout and Asparagus with Romesco Sauce

Prep time: 10 minutes | **Cook time:** 15 minutes | Makes 4

Romesco sauce is a delicious almond and red pepper blended sauce that adds hearty flavor and a beautiful aroma to fish dishes. It's the perfect complement for pink-fleshed fish like trout or salmon, but it works equally well with white fish or shellfish, too.

1 (1 pound) rainbow trout fillet, pin bones removed

1 pound asparagus, trimmed

4 tablespoons extra-virgin olive oil, divided

1 teaspoon sea salt, divided

¼ teaspoon freshly ground black pepper

1 (16-ounce) jar roasted red peppers, drained

2 tablespoons unsalted almonds

3 garlic cloves, minced

2 tablespoons red wine vinegar

1 teaspoon ground paprika

1. Preheat the oven to 400°F. Line a rimmed baking sheet with parchment paper.

2. Arrange the trout and asparagus in a single layer on the prepared sheet.

3. Drizzle with 2 tablespoons of olive oil, ½ teaspoon of salt, and the black pepper.

4. Bake in the oven until the trout is opaque and the asparagus is tender, about 15 minutes.

5. Meanwhile, in a blender, combine the red peppers, almonds, garlic cloves, red wine vinegar, paprika, remaining ½ teaspoon of sea salt, and remaining 2 tablespoons of olive oil. Blend until smooth.

6. Serve with the romesco sauce spooned over the trout and asparagus.

7. Store each component separately in the refrigerator for up to 3 days.

TIP: Adjust the consistency of the romesco sauce with a little water. For a runnier sauce, add 1 tablespoon of water at a time until reaching the desired consistency.

Per Serving (4 ounces trout, 4 ounces asparagus, 2 tablespoons romesco sauce): Calories: 339; Protein: 28g; Total fat: 20g; Total carbohydrates: 13g; Fiber: 5g; Sugars: 7g; Sodium: 567mg; Iron: 4mg

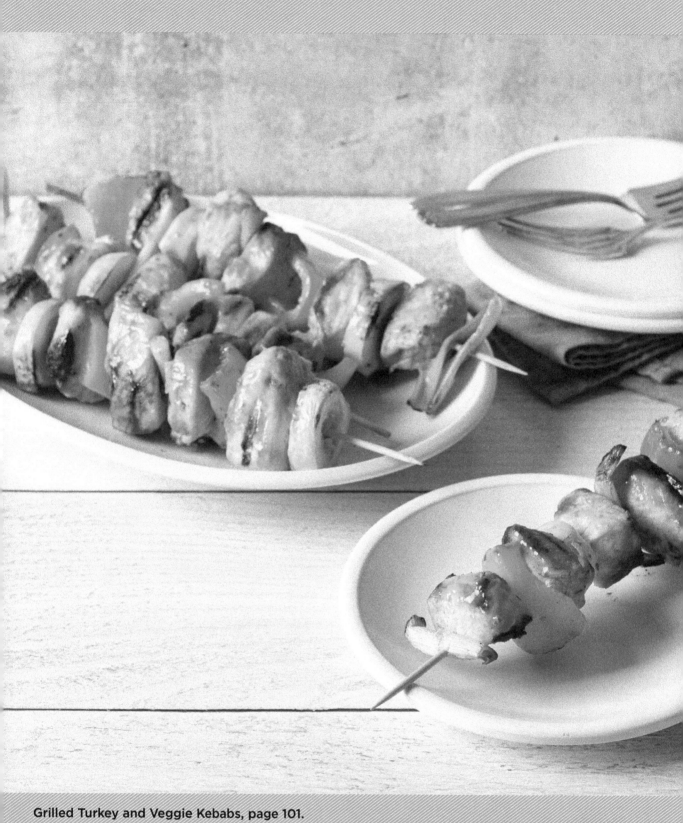

Grilled Turkey and Veggie Kebabs, page 101.

CHAPTER 8

Poultry and Meats

Chicken and Mandarin Orange Salad with Sesame Ginger Dressing

Prep time: 20 minutes | **Cook time:** 12 minutes | Makes 4

This salad hits all the right notes: It's sweet, savory, crunchy, and a bit nutty. Unlike many salads, this one is a meal-in-one and can be prepped ahead of time. The dressing is loaded with flavor but not salt, unlike many bottled dressings. It makes a flavorful and fast weeknight meal.

FOR THE DRESSING

- ¼ cup sodium-free rice wine vinegar
- 1 tablespoon sesame oil
- 1 tablespoon honey
- 2 garlic cloves, minced
- 1-inch piece fresh ginger, peeled and minced
- ¼ teaspoon kosher or sea salt

FOR THE SALAD

- 1 tablespoon canola oil
- 1 pound boneless, skinless chicken breasts
- ¼ teaspoon kosher or sea salt
- ¼ teaspoon freshly ground black pepper
- 1 large head napa cabbage, shredded
- 1 cup shredded red cabbage
- ½ cup shredded carrots
- ½ cup shelled edamame
- ½ cup sliced almonds
- 2 scallions, thinly sliced
- 1 (8 ounce) can mandarin oranges, drained

TO MAKE THE DRESSING

1. In a jar or bowl, combine the vinegar, sesame oil, honey, garlic, ginger, and salt and shake or whisk to combine. Refrigerate until ready to use.

TO MAKE THE SALAD

2. In a skillet, heat the canola oil over medium heat. Season the chicken breasts with the salt and pepper and place in the skillet. Cook for 5 to 6 minutes per side, until the chicken reaches an internal temperature of 165°F. Place on a cutting board for 5 to 10 minutes to cool and then thinly slice against the grain.

3. In a large bowl, toss the napa cabbage, red cabbage, carrots, and edamame together with the dressing. Divide into four bowls and top with the sliced chicken, almonds, scallions, and mandarin oranges.

4. If making this ahead, store the dressing, chicken, and salad separately in tightly sealed containers for up to 3 days for the chicken and the salad and for up to 5 days for the dressing. Mix before serving.

TIP: Use white vinegar instead of rice wine vinegar if needed. Use spinach instead of napa cabbage if desired.

TIP: Prep the dressing and salad ingredients ahead of time and toss together just before lunch or dinner for a simple weekday meal.

Per Serving (about 2 cups): Calories: 433; Protein: 35g; Total fat: 20g; Total carbohydrates: 32g; Fiber: 10g; Sugars: 18g; Sodium: 249mg; Iron: 3mg

Spice-Rubbed Crispy Roast Chicken

Prep time: 10 minutes | **Cook time:** 35 minutes | Makes 6

Everyone needs a quick and easy go-to chicken recipe, and this is a really good one! The combination of five spices with just a pinch of salt is the perfect blend that can be used on anything. Try it on proteins, veggies, or your favorite homemade soups. And the chicken cooks quickly because drumsticks are used, so it can be on the table in about 45 minutes.

1 teaspoon ground paprika

1 teaspoon garlic powder

½ teaspoon ground coriander

½ teaspoon ground cumin

½ teaspoon salt

¼ teaspoon cayenne pepper

6 chicken drumsticks

1 teaspoon extra-virgin olive oil

1. Preheat the oven to 400°F.

2. In a small bowl, combine the paprika, garlic powder, coriander, cumin, salt, and cayenne pepper. Rub the spices all over the chicken drumsticks.

3. In an oven-safe skillet, heat the olive oil over medium heat. Sear the chicken for 8 to 10 minutes on each side until the skin browns and becomes crisp.

4. Transfer the skillet to the oven and continue to cook for 10 to 15 minutes, until the chicken is cooked through and its juices run clear.

5. Store in the refrigerator for up to 3 days or in the freezer for up to 6 months.

TIP: Skin-on, bone-in chicken breasts work great with this rub; because they are leaner, they will take longer to cook. Plan on 2 servings per chicken breast. Sear only the skin side, and increase the baking time to 45 minutes, flipping once halfway through.

TIP: This protein-rich dish still needs veggies and carbohydrates. Add a favorite veggie-loaded soup, like Minestrone Soup (page 78), and/or Warm Barley and Squash Salad with Balsamic Vinaigrette (page 58).

Per Serving (1 drumstick): Calories: 220; Protein: 24g; Total fat: 13g; Total carbohydrates: 1g; Fiber: 0g; Sugars: 0g; Sodium: 236mg; Iron: 1mg

Grilled Turkey and Veggie Kebabs

Prep time: 20 minutes | **Cook time:** 10 minutes | Makes 4

Kebabs are a fun and efficient way to work more heart-healthy veggies into a diet. Eight (10-inch) metal kebab skewers are needed for this recipe.

1 pound turkey tenderloin, cut into 1-inch cubes

Pinch salt

⅛ teaspoon cayenne pepper

1 yellow summer squash, cut into ½-inch slices

1 orange bell pepper, seeded, ribs removed, and cut into 1-inch cubes

1 red bell pepper, seeded, ribs removed, and cut into 1-inch cubes

3 scallions, cut into 2-inch pieces

2 tablespoons honey

2 tablespoons apple juice

2 tablespoons lemon juice

1 tablespoon butter

1 tablespoon low-sodium mustard

1 teaspoon dried oregano

1. Preheat the grill or grill pan to medium heat.

2. Put the turkey cubes on a plate and sprinkle with the salt and cayenne pepper.

3. Thread the turkey cubes, alternating with the squash, orange bell pepper, red bell pepper, and scallions, onto kebab skewers.

4. In a small saucepan, combine the honey, apple juice, lemon juice, and butter. Heat over low heat until the honey melts and the mixture is smooth, about 2 minutes. Stir in the mustard and oregano.

5. Place the kebabs on the hot grill and brush with some of the honey mixture. Cover and grill for 4 minutes.

6. Uncover, turn the kebabs, and brush with more of the honey mixture. Cover and grill for 3 minutes more.

7. Uncover the grill and turn the kebabs, brushing with the remaining honey mixture, and cook until the turkey reaches an internal temperature of 165°F, 2 to 3 minutes longer. Use all of the honey mixture; if any is left, discard it.

8. Store in individual servings in zip-top bags in the refrigerator for up to 3 days or in the freezer for up to 6 months.

Per Serving (about 2 kebabs): Calories: 225; Protein: 28g; Total fat: 5g; Total carbohydrates: 17g; Fiber: 2g; Sugars: 14g; Sodium: 239mg; Iron: 2mg

Avgolemono Soup with Chicken Meatballs

Prep time: 10 minutes | **Cook time:** 25 minutes | Makes 6

This lemony soup has the nice bite of garlic, bright acid from the lemons, and rich, tender, aromatic chicken meatballs. It's a delicious and satisfying soup that packs, travels, and reheats well, making it a perfect dinner with leftovers that can be enjoyed for lunch the next day.

1 pound ground chicken breast

10 garlic cloves minced, divided

2 tablespoons Italian seasoning

1 teaspoon sea salt, divided

½ teaspoon freshly ground black pepper, divided

2 tablespoons extra-virgin olive oil

1 onion, chopped

3 carrots, chopped

6 cups low-sodium vegetable broth

Juice of 3 lemons

6 eggs

2 cups baby spinach

1. In a mixing bowl, combine the ground chicken breast with half of the garlic, the Italian seasoning, ½ teaspoon of sea salt, and ¼ teaspoon of pepper. Roll into 1-inch meatballs and set aside.

2. In a large pot, heat the olive oil over medium-high heat until it shimmers. Add the onion and carrots and cook, stirring occasionally, until soft, about 5 minutes.

3. Add the remaining garlic and cook, stirring constantly, for 30 seconds.

4. Add the vegetable broth, remaining ½ teaspoon of salt, and remaining ¼ teaspoon of pepper. Bring to a boil.

5. Carefully add the meatballs to the boiling broth. Bring the soup back to boiling and reduce the heat to medium. Cook, stirring occasionally, until the meatballs are cooked through, about 20 minutes.

6. Turn the heat back up to medium-high. In a small bowl, whisk together the lemon juice and eggs.

7. Add a few tablespoons of hot broth to the eggs, 1 tablespoon at a time, whisking and adding slowly to temper the eggs so they don't harden in the soup.

8. Now, stirring the soup constantly, pour the egg and lemon mixture back into the soup.

9. Stir in the spinach and cook, stirring, just until softened, about 1 minute more.

10. Store in single-serving containers in the refrigerator for up to 3 days or in the freezer for up to 6 months.

TIP: For an even brighter citrus flavor, stir in ½ teaspoon of grated lemon zest just before serving.

Per Serving (about 1½ cups and about 5 meatballs): Calories: 254; Protein: 21g; Total fat: 15g; Total carbohydrates: 9g; Fiber: 2g; Sugars: 3g; Sodium: 341mg; Iron: 2mg

Baked Turkey Kofta Meatballs with Tricolored Peppers

Prep time: 15 minutes | **Cook time:** 30 minutes | Makes 4

The combination of spices for this savory dish is traditional in Mediterranean and Middle Eastern cuisine. It makes the kofta meatballs super fragrant and flavorful.

3 bell peppers in different colors, seeded, ribs removed, and thinly sliced

2 tablespoons extra-virgin olive oil

1 yellow onion, grated

1 pound ground turkey breast

4 garlic cloves, minced

1 tablespoon ground coriander

1 teaspoon ground cumin

1 teaspoon ground paprika

½ teaspoon ground cinnamon

½ teaspoon ground ginger

½ teaspoon sea salt

¼ teaspoon ground allspice

1. Preheat the oven to 375°F. Line two rimmed baking sheets with parchment paper.

2. Spread the bell peppers in a single layer on the prepared baking sheets and drizzle with the olive oil.

3. Wring out the grated onion in a tea towel over the sink to remove water.

4. In a medium bowl, add the onion, turkey, garlic, coriander, cumin, paprika, cinnamon, ginger, salt, and allspice. Mix well and form into 1-inch meatballs.

5. Put the meatballs on top of the bell peppers.

6. Bake in the oven until the meatballs reach an internal temperature of 165°F, about 30 minutes.

7. The meatballs freeze well and are excellent reheated and served with salads, soups, or other veggies. Store them in single servings (about five meatballs) in zip-top bags in the freezer for up to 6 months (or in the refrigerator for up to 3 days).

TIP: Try cooking these meatballs on the grill. Divide into eight portions and wrap each around a metal skewer. Brush with olive oil and grill for about 30 minutes, turning occasionally.

Per Serving (about ½ cup peppers and 5 meatballs): Calories: 288; Protein: 23g; Total fat: 17g; Total carbohydrates: 13g; Fiber: 2g; Sugars: 1g; Sodium: 230mg; Iron: 3mg

Ground Turkey and Veggie Stir-Fry

Prep time: 10 minutes | **Cook time:** 15 minutes | Makes 4

Stir-fries make excellent weeknight meals because they are quick cooking and bursting with flavor. It's also a great way to use seasonal veggies or leftover vegetables. When served over cooked brown rice, it's a hearty and satisfying meal.

2 tablespoons extra-virgin olive oil

1 pound ground turkey

2 carrots, sliced

1 bunch scallions, sliced

2 cups broccoli florets

1 red bell pepper, seeded, ribs removed, and chopped

3 garlic cloves, minced

2 teaspoons grated ginger

1 tablespoon reduced-sodium soy sauce or tamari

Juice of 1 orange

2 cups cooked brown rice

1. In a large nonstick skillet, heat the olive oil over medium-high heat until it shimmers.

2. Add the turkey and cook, crumbling with a spoon, until it browns, about 5 minutes.

3. Add the carrots, scallions, broccoli, and bell pepper. Cook, stirring, until the vegetables are crisp-tender, 5 to 7 minutes.

4. Add the garlic and ginger and cook, stirring constantly, for 30 seconds.

5. Add the soy sauce and orange juice. Cook, stirring, for 3 minutes more.

6. Serve spooned over the rice.

7. Store in 1½-cup servings in the refrigerator for up to 3 days or in the freezer for up to 6 months. Store the rice and stir-fry separately.

TIP: Other veggies that work well in this stir-fry include shredded cabbage, pea pods, and green beans.

Per Serving (about 1½ cups and ½ cup rice): Calories: 387; Protein: 26g; Total fat: 17g; Total carbohydrates: 32g; Fiber: 4g; Sugars: 5g; Sodium: 387mg; Iron: 3mg

Mediterranean Chicken Skillet

Prep time: 15 minutes | **Cook time:** 20 minutes | Makes 4

This is a quick skillet meal that's similar to a stir-fry. It's delicious on its own, or it can be served over ½ cup of cooked whole-wheat pasta for a heartier meal.

2 tablespoons extra-virgin olive oil

1 pound boneless, skinless chicken breast, sliced

1 red onion, sliced

1 red bell pepper, seeded, ribs removed, and sliced

½ cup sliced black olives

1 pint cherry tomatoes, halved

1 (14-ounce) can artichoke hearts, drained and quartered

1 tablespoon Italian seasoning

3 garlic cloves, minced

Juice and grated zest of 1 lemon

½ teaspoon sea salt

1. In a large nonstick skillet, heat the olive oil over medium-high heat until it shimmers.

2. Add the chicken and cook, stirring occasionally, until it is opaque and cooked through, about 7 minutes. Use tongs to remove the chicken from the skillet and set aside on a platter, tented with foil to keep warm.

3. In the same pan, add the onion and bell pepper. Cook, stirring occasionally, until the vegetables begin to soften, about 5 minutes.

4. Add the olives, tomatoes, artichoke hearts, and Italian seasoning. Cook, stirring occasionally, for 3 minutes more.

5. Add the garlic and cook, stirring constantly, for 30 seconds.

6. Return the chicken to the pan along with any juices that have collected on the platter. Add the lemon juice and zest and salt. Cook, stirring, for 1 minute more.

7. Store in about 1-cup servings in the refrigerator for up to 3 days or in the freezer in individual servings for up to 6 months.

TIP: When grating lemon zest, lightly grate so only the yellow part comes off the lemon.

Per Serving (about 1 cup): Calories: 279; Protein: 29g; Total fat: 11g; Total carbohydrates: 18g; Fiber: 9g; Sugars: 5g; Sodium: 383mg; Iron: 2mg

Turkey Tapenade Burgers

Prep time: 15 minutes | **Cook time:** 10 minutes | Makes 4

Tapenade is an olive spread that's brimming with healthy omega-3 oils and delicious olive flavor. A little goes a long way, but it's delicious on burgers like these, on sandwiches, or even as a dip for veggies. Want to fancy it up? Use Kalamata olives from the salad bar in place of the black olives for a slightly sweeter, richer olive flavor.

1 pound ground turkey breast

1 garlic clove, minced

1 tablespoon Dijon mustard

½ teaspoon sea salt

1 tablespoon extra-virgin olive oil

2 whole-wheat pitas, cut in half

4 servings Tapenade (page 130)

4 tomato slices

1 cup arugula

4 thin slices red onion

1. In a large bowl, combine the turkey breast, garlic, mustard, and salt. Mix well.

2. Form into four patties.

3. In a large nonstick skillet, heat the olive oil over medium-high heat.

4. Add the burgers and cook until the turkey reaches an internal temperature of 165°F, about 5 minutes per side.

5. Spread the inside of the pitas with the tapenade. Place the patties in the pita halves and add the tomato slices, arugula, and red onion slices.

6. Store the turkey patties, tapenade, pitas, and toppings separately. Store the turkey patties in the refrigerator for up to 3 days or in the freezer for up to 6 months. Tapenade will keep in the refrigerator for up to 1 week.

TIP: Warm pitas are even better than room-temperature pitas! Place the pitas on a baking sheet in a 325°F oven for about 5 minutes to warm them before serving.

Per Serving (about 1 cup): Calories: 349; Protein: 25g; Total fat: 19g; Total carbohydrates: 22g; Fiber: 4g; Sugars: 1g; Sodium: 516mg; Iron: 4mg

Pesto-Stuffed Chicken Roulade

Prep time: 15 minutes | **Cook time:** 30 minutes | Makes 4

Chicken by itself can be a little bland, but when stuffed with a zippy pesto and some spin-ach, it has a tremendous amount of flavor and color. Fair warning: This is going to smell great as it roasts in the oven and will make any mouth water.

4 boneless, skinless chicken breasts

½ teaspoon sea salt

¼ teaspoon freshly ground black pepper

1 cup Basil Pesto (page 124), divided

3 cups baby spinach

2 red bell peppers, seeded, ribs removed, and very thinly sliced

1. Preheat the oven to 375°F. Line a rimmed baking sheet with parchment paper.

2. Place each chicken breast between two pieces of parchment paper or plastic wrap and pound to an even ¼-inch thickness.

3. Season the chicken breasts with salt and black pepper. Spread each with ¼ cup of pesto.

4. Place the spinach on the pesto in a thin layer and then place red bell pepper slices on top.

5. Roll tightly and tie with kitchen twine. Place on the parchment paper–lined baking sheet.

6. Bake in the oven until the chicken reaches an internal temperature of 165°F, about 30 minutes, flipping about halfway through cooking.

7. Store these individually plastic wrapped in the refrigerator for up to 3 days or in the freezer for up to 6 months.

TIP: These chicken breasts are a great source of both protein and veggies. Feel free to serve them alongside an additional veggie, such as Garlicky Green Beans (page 67).

Per Serving (about 1 breast): Calories: 466; Protein: 33g; Total fat: 33g; Total carbohydrates: 7g; Fiber: 2g; Sugars: 3g; Sodium: 484mg; Iron: 1mg

Mustard and Herb Pork Tenderloin

Prep time: 10 minutes | **Cook time:** 30 minutes | Makes 4

The mustard and fresh herb crust on the outside of this pork tenderloin makes for a mouthwatering main dish. The root veggies are cooked right in the sheet pan along with the pork, so it's a single sheet pan dinner that's fast, easy, and flavorful.

2 tablespoons extra-virgin olive oil

1 pound baby red potatoes, quartered

6 carrots, coarsely chopped

2 red onions, cut into 8 pieces

1 teaspoon sea salt, divided

½ teaspoon black pepper, divided

¼ cup chopped fresh parsley

2 tablespoons Dijon mustard

2 tablespoons chopped fresh rosemary

3 garlic cloves, minced

1 pound pork tenderloin

1. Preheat the oven to 425°F. Line a rimmed baking sheet with parchment paper.

2. In a large bowl, toss the olive oil with the potatoes, carrots, onions, ½ teaspoon of salt, and ¼ teaspoon of pepper. Spread in a single layer on the rimmed baking sheet.

3. In a small bowl, mix the parsley, mustard, rosemary, garlic, remaining ½ teaspoon of salt, and the remaining ¼ teaspoon pepper.

4. Spread the mustard mixture evenly over the pork tenderloin and place it with the vegetables on the baking sheet.

5. Roast in the oven until the veggies are browned and tender and the tenderloin reaches an internal temperature of 160°F, about 30 minutes. Allow to rest for 5 minutes before cutting into four slices.

6. Store the sliced pork separately from the roasted root veggies. Both will keep in the refrigerator for up to 3 days.

TIP: You can replace the potatoes with Brussels sprouts. Trim and quarter 1 pound of Brussels sprouts instead of potatoes and place, cut-side down, on the baking sheet.

Per Serving (about 4 ounces pork and about 1 cup veggies): Calories: 345; Protein: 28g; Total fat: 11g; Total carbohydrates: 33g; Fiber: 6g; Sugars: 8g; Sodium: 524mg; Iron: 3mg

Patty Melt Soup

Prep time: 10 minutes | **Cook time:** 45 minutes | Makes 6

This soup tastes just like a classic American patty melt burger. With deep flavors of caramelized onion and seasoned with caraway seeds (found in the spice aisle), this soup is sure to satisfy any craving for American diner food in a creative way.

2 tablespoons
extra-virgin olive oil

2 yellow onions,
thinly sliced

1 pound extra-lean
ground beef

3 garlic cloves, minced

6 cups low-sodium
vegetable broth

3 carrots, chopped

1 tablespoon dried
mustard powder

1 teaspoon ground
caraway seeds

½ teaspoon sea salt

¼ teaspoon freshly
ground black pepper

1. In a large pot, heat the olive oil over medium-high heat until it shimmers. Add the onions and cook, stirring occasionally, for 3 minutes until they begin to soften.

2. Reduce the heat to medium-low and continue to cook the onions, stirring occasionally, until they are golden brown, about 25 minutes more.

3. Remove the onions from the pan and set aside. Add the ground beef and return the heat to medium-high. Cook, crumbling, until the beef is browned, about 5 minutes.

4. Add the garlic and cook, stirring constantly, for 30 seconds.

5. Add the vegetable broth, carrots, mustard powder, caraway seeds, salt, and pepper. Bring to a boil and reduce the heat to medium.

6. Simmer until the carrots soften, about 10 minutes more. Return the onions to the pan and cook until heated through, about 1 minute.

7. Store in 1½-cup servings in the refrigerator for up to 3 days or in the freezer for up to 6 months.

Per Serving (about 1½ cups): Calories: 175; Protein: 17g; Total fat: 9g; Total carbohydrates: 7g; Fiber: 2g; Sugars: 3g; Sodium: 170mg; Iron: 2mg

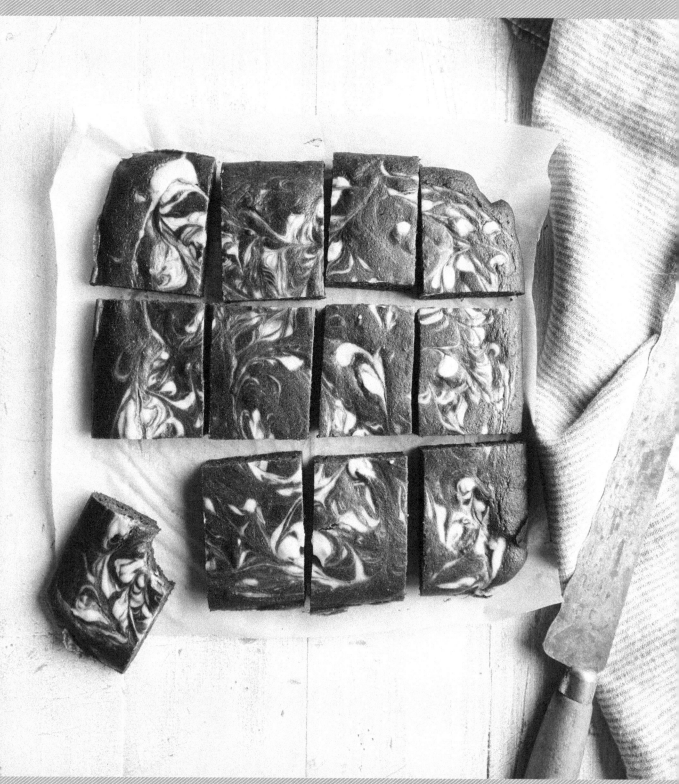

Cream Cheese Swirl Brownies, page 115.

CHAPTER 9

Snacks and Treats

Oatmeal Dark Chocolate Chip Peanut Butter Cookies

Prep time: 15 minutes | **Cook time:** 10 minutes | Makes 24

These chocolate chip cookies include wholesome ingredients like peanut butter, rolled oats, and dark chocolate chips. Bake them for 8 minutes for a chewier, soft cookie or for 10 minutes for a crispier cookie. Either way, they make the perfect guilt-free dessert.

1½ cups natural creamy peanut butter

½ cup dark brown sugar

2 large eggs

1 cup old-fashioned rolled oats

1 teaspoon baking soda

½ teaspoon kosher or sea salt

½ cup dark chocolate chips

1. Preheat the oven to 350°F. Line a baking sheet with parchment paper.

2. In a bowl, cream together the peanut butter and brown sugar until smooth.

3. Add the eggs and mix well.

4. Add the oats, baking soda, and salt. Stir until well combined. Fold in the chocolate chips.

5. Using a small cookie scoop or teaspoon, place globs of the cookie dough on the baking sheet, about 2 inches apart. Bake for 8 to 10 minutes depending on the preferred level of doneness.

6. Store, tightly sealed, at room temperature for up to 1 week or in a zip-top bag in the freezer for up to 6 months.

TIP: Try raisins instead of the chocolate chips. For a gluten-free version, choose gluten-free oats.

TIP: For a fluffier cookie, refrigerate the dough for 30 minutes before baking.

Per Serving (about 1 cookie): Calories: 153; Protein: 5g; Total fat: 11g; Total carbohydrates: 11g; Fiber: 2g; Sugars: 6g; Sodium: 120mg; Iron: 1mg

Cream Cheese Swirl Brownies

Prep time: 10 minutes | **Cook time:** 20 minutes | Makes 12

Brownies are the ultimate crowd-pleaser. This version is moist with deep chocolate flavors and the gooey intensity that makes brownies so satisfying. So the next time you need a chocolate fix, try one of these brownies. They aren't overloaded with highly processed ingredients or sweeteners, but they're so rich, those won't be missed.

2 eggs

¼ cup unsweetened applesauce

¼ cup coconut oil, melted

3 tablespoons pure maple syrup, divided

¼ cup unsweetened cocoa powder

¼ cup coconut flour

1 teaspoon baking powder

¼ teaspoon salt

2 tablespoons low-fat cream cheese

1. Preheat the oven to 350°F. Grease an 8 x 8-inch baking dish.

2. In a large mixing bowl, beat the eggs, applesauce, coconut oil, and 2 tablespoons of maple syrup.

3. Stir in the cocoa powder and coconut flour and mix well. Sprinkle the baking powder and salt evenly over the surface and mix well to incorporate. Transfer the mixture to the prepared baking dish.

4. In a small, microwave-safe bowl, microwave the cream cheese for 10 to 20 seconds until softened. Add the remaining 1 tablespoon of maple syrup and mix to combine.

5. Drop the cream cheese onto the batter, and use a toothpick or chopstick to swirl it on the surface. Bake for 20 minutes, until a toothpick inserted in the center comes out clean. Cool and cut into twelve squares.

6. Store in an airtight container in the refrigerator for up to 5 days.

TIP: Sprinkle ½ cup of chopped walnuts on the top before baking to make a heartier treat.

Per Serving (1 brownie): Calories: 84; Protein: 2g; Total fat: 6g; Total carbohydrates: 6g; Fiber: 2g; Sugars: 4g; Sodium: 93mg; Iron: 1mg

Lemon-Garlic Kale Chips

Prep time: 5 minutes | **Cook time:** 15 minutes | Makes 4

Kale chips are an excellent substitute for potato chips. Like potatoes, kale itself does not have a strong flavor and relies on complementary flavors. The garlic powder and lemon juice give these chips enough flavor that salt won't need to be added, and baking the kale gives it a crisp texture similar to traditional potato chips.

1 (16-ounce) bag torn kale leaves

2 tablespoons extra-virgin olive oil

1 tablespoon garlic powder

Grated zest and juice of ½ lemon

1. Preheat the oven to 300°F. Line a baking sheet with aluminum foil.

2. In a large bowl, combine the kale, olive oil, and garlic powder. Add the lemon zest and lemon juice and toss to coat. Arrange the kale in a single layer on the prepared baking sheet.

3. Bake for about 15 minutes, until the kale is crisp but not burnt.

4. Store leftovers in an airtight container at room temperature for up to 1 week.

TIP: Make these chips spicy by adding a pinch of cayenne pepper to the mix.

Per Serving (about 1 cup): Calories: 125; Protein: 5g; Total fat: 8g; Total carbohydrates: 12g; Fiber: 4g; Sugars: 3g; Sodium: 45mg; Iron: 2mg

Baba Ghanoush and Veggies

Prep time: 5 minutes | **Cook time:** 30 minutes | Makes 4

Baba ghanoush is similar to hummus, but eggplant is used instead of chickpeas. Slice the eggplant before cooking to save time in the oven and roast the eggplant until the slices are soft enough to mash.

4 servings Oven-Roasted Eggplant Slices (page 63)

¼ cup tahini

Juice of ½ lemon

2 tablespoons extra-virgin olive oil

2 garlic cloves, minced

½ teaspoon ground cumin

½ teaspoon ground paprika

½ teaspoon sea salt

4 carrots, cut into sticks

1. Place the hot eggplant slices in a colander in the sink for 20 minutes to allow excess liquid to drain. Using a sharp knife, trim away the peel. Chop the eggplant and put it in a large bowl.

2. Add the tahini, lemon juice, olive oil, garlic, cumin, paprika, and salt. Mash with a fork until the eggplant is mashed, and then stir well.

3. Serve warm or chilled with the carrots for dipping.

4. Store in the refrigerator for up to 5 days.

TIP: The best way to get evenly minced garlic is to put it through a garlic press.

Per Serving (about ¼ cup and 1 carrot): Calories: 200; Protein: 4g; Total fat: 15g; Total carbohydrates: 15g; Fiber: 6g; Sugars: 6g; Sodium: 207mg; Iron: 2mg

Hummus and Bell Peppers

Prep time: 5 minutes | Makes 4

Canned chickpeas make this traditional Mediterranean dip fast and easy. This is not only tasty served as a dip for bell peppers, but it's equally delicious served as a side with a kebab, meatball, or even grilled chicken. This recipe is for a traditional hummus, but you can add a roasted red bell pepper for a bit of sweetness and color.

1 (14-ounce) can chickpeas, drained

2 tablespoons tahini

Juice of 1 lemon

Grated zest of ½ lemon

2 tablespoons extra-virgin olive oil, plus more for drizzling

1 garlic clove, finely minced

½ teaspoon sea salt

Ground paprika, for garnish

2 bell peppers, seeded, ribs removed, and sliced

1. In a blender, combine the chickpeas, tahini, lemon juice and zest, olive oil, garlic (to taste), and salt.

2. Blend until smooth. Put into a serving bowl. Drizzle with a little olive oil and sprinkle with paprika.

3. Serve with the sliced bell peppers for dipping.

4. Store tightly sealed in the refrigerator for up to 5 days.

TIP: For a little extra flavor and texture, sprinkle 1 tablespoon of toasted sesame seeds or pine nuts on the hummus.

Per Serving (about ¼ cup and ½ bell pepper): Calories: 234; Protein: 8g; Total fat: 13g; Total carbohydrates: 25g; Fiber: 6g; Sugars: 3g; Sodium: 161mg; Iron: 3mg

Fruit with Tahini Dip

Prep time: 5 minutes | Makes 4

One of the great things about tahini is that it's delicious in both sweet and savory applications. This version combines orange, cinnamon, and honey with tahini and yogurt for a creamy, complex dip that pairs beautifully with berries or sliced tree fruits such as apples or pears. It makes a delicious snack or dessert.

¼ cup tahini

¼ cup plain Greek yogurt

Grated zest and juice of ½ orange

½ teaspoon ground cinnamon

½ teaspoon ground ginger

2 tablespoons honey

2 tablespoons chopped walnuts

4 apples, cored and sliced, or fruit of choice

1. In a medium bowl, whisk together the tahini, yogurt, orange juice and zest, cinnamon, ginger, and honey.

2. Sprinkle with the walnuts.

3. Serve with the sliced apples for dipping.

4. Store in the refrigerator for up to 3 days.

TIP: If more ginger is desired, chop 2 tablespoons of candied ginger and stir it in for texture and additional flavor.

Per Serving (about 2 tablespoons dip and 1 apple): Calories: 255; Protein: 4g; Total fat: 11g; Total carbohydrates: 40g; Fiber: 6g; Sugars: 29g; Sodium: 27mg; Iron: 2mg

Crispy Roasted Mushroom Slices

Prep time: 10 minutes | **Cook time:** 50 minutes | Makes 4

If the earthy, umami flavor of mushrooms is pleasing, these simple chips are sure to hit the spot for a snack food. They're super simple; the majority of the time is spent in the oven because they take some time to dry and crisp.

8 ounces cremini mushrooms, thinly sliced

2 tablespoons extra-virgin olive oil

½ teaspoon sea salt

1. Preheat the oven to 325°F. Line two baking sheets with parchment paper.

2. Place the mushroom slices in a single layer on the prepared sheets. Brush with the olive oil and sprinkle with the sea salt.

3. Bake in the oven until the mushrooms are crisp, about 50 minutes.

4. Store in a zip-top bag at room temperature for up to 5 days.

TIP: Don't wash the mushrooms; they're like sponges and will get waterlogged. Instead, clean them with a dry mushroom brush or dry paper towel, wiping away any dirt.

Per Serving (about ¼ cup): Calories: 72; Protein: 1g; Total fat: 7g; Total carbohydrates: 2g; Fiber: 0g; Sugars: 1g; Sodium: 149mg; Iron: 0mg

Whole-Wheat Pita Chips

Prep time: 10 minutes | **Cook time:** 12 minutes | Makes 4

For something crispy and hearty to bring dip to your mouth, pita chips are the perfect vehicle. These lightly seasoned chips are solid and structured so they won't crumble under the weight of a dip. They're not as fatty or salty as commercial chips, so they're perfect for snacking.

4 whole-wheat pita rounds, cut into 8 wedges each

2 tablespoons extra-virgin olive oil

½ teaspoon sea salt

½ teaspoon garlic powder

1. Preheat the oven to 350°F. Line two baking sheets with parchment paper.

2. Spread the pita wedges on the baking sheets in a single layer.

3. In a small bowl, whisk together the olive oil, salt, and garlic powder. Brush on the chips.

4. Bake in the oven until browned and crisp, 10 to 12 minutes.

5. Cool completely before serving or storing.

6. Store in a zip-top bag at room temperature for up to 5 days.

TIP: Flavor-wise, these chips are easy to customize. Mix ½ teaspoon of flavored oil, such as truffle oil or sesame oil, in with the olive oil or add other spices in place of garlic powder, such as chili powder or smoked paprika.

Per Serving (about 8 wedges): Calories: 231; Protein: 6g; Total fat: 8g; Total carbohydrates: 35g; Fiber: 5g; Sugars: 1g; Sodium: 330mg; Iron: 2mg

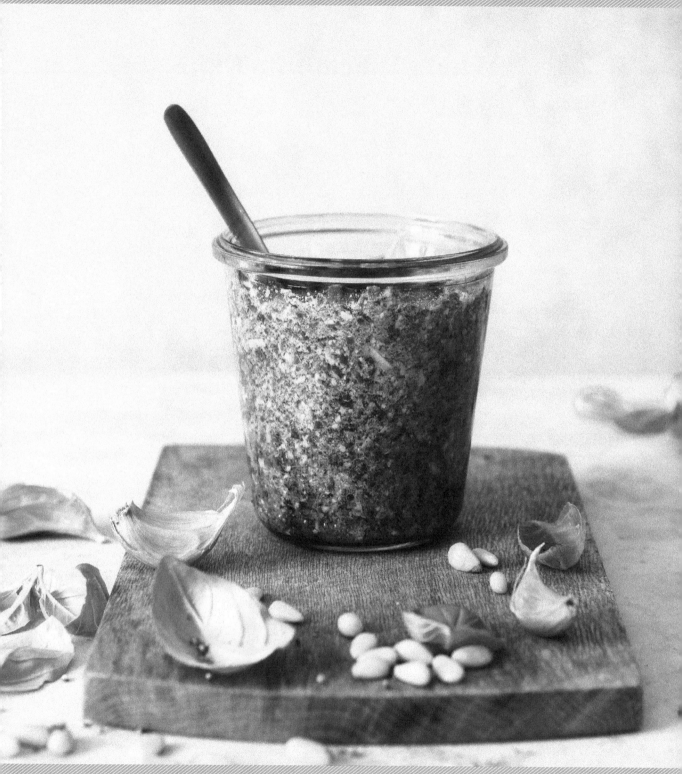

Basil Pesto, page 124.

CHAPTER 10

Homemade Staples

Basil Pesto

Prep time: 10 minutes | Makes 3½ cups

Pesto is a quintessential northern Italian sauce and condiment full of fresh basil. Not only is it delicious, it is considered heart healthy because it's made with superfoods like olive oil, nuts, and garlic. A little goes a long way, though, as it's loaded with flavor but is also calorie-dense.

1 cup fresh basil leaves

1 cup fresh baby spinach leaves

½ cup freshly grated Parmesan cheese

½ cup extra-virgin olive oil

¼ cup pine nuts

4 garlic cloves, peeled

¼ teaspoon kosher or sea salt

¼ teaspoon freshly ground black pepper

1. In the bowl of a food processor, combine the basil, spinach, Parmesan cheese, olive oil, pine nuts, garlic, salt, and pepper and process until a paste forms, scraping down the sides of the bowl with a spatula as needed. Taste and adjust the seasoning, if necessary.

2. Store in airtight containers in the refrigerator for up to 5 days, or in the freezer for up to 2 months and thaw as needed. Or divide the pesto into ice cube trays, seal in a zip-top bag, and store in the freezer for up to 2 months. Pop pesto cubes out of the ice cube tray as needed.

TIP: Use nutritional yeast instead of Parmesan cheese to make this recipe vegan.

TIP: Try any seeds or nuts, like pepitas, walnuts, or almonds, instead of pine nuts, if desired.

Per Serving (¼ cup): Calories: 102; Protein: 2g; Total fat: 10g; Total carbohydrates: 1g; Fiber: 0g; Sugars: 0g; Sodium: 89mg; Iron: 0mg

Homemade Turkey Breakfast Sausage

Prep time: 10 minutes | **Cook time:** 10 minutes | Makes 8

Most people don't realize that making sausage at home is incredibly easy. This breakfast sausage can be made with common spices you already have in the cupboard. It's impressive how simple it is to replicate the flavor of the store-bought versions, only without the unwanted hidden sugar and salt.

1 pound lean ground turkey

½ teaspoon salt

½ teaspoon ground sage

½ teaspoon dried thyme

½ teaspoon freshly ground black pepper

¼ teaspoon ground fennel seeds

1 teaspoon extra-virgin olive oil

1. In a large mixing bowl, combine the turkey, salt, sage, thyme, pepper, and fennel seeds. Mix well.

2. Shape the meat into eight small, round patties. Use this in recipes or cook as noted in the remaining steps and store for later.

3. In a skillet, heat the olive oil over medium-high heat. Cook the patties in the skillet for 3 to 4 minutes on each side until browned and cooked through.

4. Serve warm, or store in an airtight container in the refrigerator for up to 3 days or in the freezer for up to 1 month.

TIP: If using the turkey sausage for the Sweet Potato, Onion, and Turkey Sausage Hash (page 45), skip steps 2 and 3, and add the bulk sausage to the pan when called for in the recipe.

Per Serving (1 patty): Calories: 91; Protein: 11g; Total fat: 5g; Total carbohydrates: 0g; Fiber: 0g; Sugars: 0g; Sodium: 185mg; Iron: 1mg

Greek Lemon Vinaigrette

Prep time: 10 minutes | Makes 4

This is a simple and flavorful vinaigrette with bright acid from the lemon juice, along with aromatic garlic and savory oregano. This can be used in the Greek Salad (page 61), or toss it with greens or raw or cooked veggies. It's also a delicious marinade for poultry or fish to add more flavor.

¼ cup red wine vinegar

3 garlic cloves, finely minced

2 tablespoons freshly squeezed lemon juice

2 tablespoons dried oregano

1 teaspoon Dijon mustard

¼ teaspoon sea salt

⅛ teaspoon freshly ground black pepper

¼ cup extra-virgin olive oil

1. In a small bowl, whisk together the red wine vinegar, garlic, lemon juice, oregano, mustard, salt, and pepper.

2. Pour in the olive oil in a thin stream, whisking constantly.

3. Store in a bottle in the refrigerator for up to 2 weeks. Shake before using.

TIP: Hoping to avoid making a dirty bowl? Put all the ingredients in a jar or bottle and shake until they are well mixed and emulsified.

Per Serving (about 2 tablespoons): Calories: 132; Protein: 0g; Total fat: 14g; Total carbohydrates: 2g; Fiber: 1g; Sugars: 0g; Sodium: 94mg; Iron: 1mg

Mango Salsa

Prep time: 10 minutes, plus 20 minutes to rest | Makes 4

This simple salsa fresca (fresh salsa) has bright and complex flavors that are delicious as a cracker dip and are even tastier as a condiment. It can be used on tacos or sandwiches, or as a topping for freshly grilled fish. With a little sweet and a little heat, it's sure to become a family favorite.

1 cup chopped
   fresh mango

½ red onion, diced

¼ cup chopped fresh
   cilantro

1 jalapeño pepper,
   seeded, ribs removed,
   and minced

1 garlic clove,
   finely minced

Juice of 1 lime

½ teaspoon sea salt

1. In a small bowl, combine the mango, onion, cilantro, jalapeño, garlic, lime juice, and salt. Mix well.

2. Allow to sit at room temperature for about 20 minutes for the flavors to blend.

3. While this is best fresh, it can be stored tightly sealed in the refrigerator for up to 5 days.

TIP: For a more traditional salsa fresca, replace the mango with fresh tomato.

Per Serving (about ¼ cup): Calories: 35; Protein: 1g; Total fat: 0g; Total carbohydrates: 9g; Fiber: 1g; Sugars: 6g; Sodium: 147mg; Iron: 0mg

Guacamole

Prep time: 10 minutes | Makes 4

Fresh guacamole is creamy and rich with bright hints of heat and acid. It's also super easy to prepare. Serve it on whole-wheat toast as a breakfast, enjoy it with some eggs, use it as a sandwich spread, enjoy it as a veggie dip, or serve it on Southwestern favorites like tacos or burritos.

1 avocado, peeled, pitted, and cubed

Juice of ½ lime

1 garlic clove, minced

¼ teaspoon sea salt

¼ red onion, finely minced

½ jalapeño pepper, seeded, ribs removed, and minced

2 tablespoons chopped fresh cilantro

1. In a small bowl, combine the avocado, lime juice, garlic, and salt.

2. Use a fork to mash the avocado and other ingredients until the desired consistency.

3. Stir in the onion, jalapeño, and cilantro.

4. Store in a small bowl or container. Place a layer of plastic wrap directly on the surface of the guacamole (rather than stretched over the top where air will be trapped) to keep it from browning, and then seal the container. It will keep this way in the refrigerator for up to 3 days.

TIP: Choose avocadoes that are relatively soft. When pressing the avocado with a finger, it should have some give but not be mushy.

Per Serving (about ¼ cup): Calories: 86; Protein: 1g; Total fat: 7g; Total carbohydrates: 6g; Fiber: 4g; Sugars: 1g; Sodium: 82mg; Iron: 0mg

Garlicky Cucumber Yogurt Sauce

Prep time: 10 minutes, plus 30 minutes to chill | Makes 4

Cucumber yogurt sauce, also called tzatziki, *is a delicious Mediterranean condiment with a fresh and savory flavor. It's delicious on salads, poultry, fish, and meat, or served as a dip for veggies or chips, such as Whole-Wheat Pita Chips (page 121). Don't skip the step of draining the cucumbers, or the dip will become too watery.*

1 medium cucumber, grated on a box grater

1 cup plain Greek yogurt

Juice and grated zest of ½ lemon

1 tablespoon extra-virgin olive oil

2 garlic cloves, minced

1 tablespoon chopped fresh dill (optional)

¼ teaspoon sea salt

⅛ teaspoon freshly ground black pepper

1. Put the cucumber in a colander in the sink and allow it to drain for about 30 minutes.

2. In a bowl, whisk together the yogurt, lemon juice and zest, olive oil, garlic, dill, salt, and pepper until smooth.

3. Fold in the cucumber.

4. Refrigerate for about 30 minutes before serving.

5. Store tightly sealed in the refrigerator for up to 3 days.

TIP: If fresh dill isn't available, try ½ teaspoon of dried dill instead.

Per Serving (about ¼ cup): Calories: 82; Protein: 3g; Total fat: 5g; Total carbohydrates: 7g; Fiber: 0g; Sugars: 4g; Sodium: 108mg; Iron: 0mg

Tapenade

Prep time: 10 minutes, plus 30 minutes to chill | Makes 4

Tapenade is a rich and flavorful addition to any menu, and it's loaded with nutritious, anti-inflammatory ingredients like olives. It is a multi-use condiment that can be spread on toast, crackers, or sandwiches, used as a condiment for fish or poultry, or as a dip for veggies.

½ cup pitted black olives, finely chopped

¼ cup fresh basil leaves, minced

3 garlic cloves, minced

1 tablespoon extra-virgin olive oil

1 teaspoon Dijon mustard

1 teaspoon Italian seasoning

1 teaspoon red wine vinegar

1 teaspoon grated lemon zest

¼ teaspoon sea salt

⅛ teaspoon freshly ground black pepper

Pinch red pepper flakes

1. In a blender, combine the black olives, basil, garlic, olive oil, mustard, Italian seasoning, vinegar, lemon zest, salt, black pepper, and red pepper flakes. Pulse for 10 one-second pulses to blend.

2. Allow to rest in the refrigerator for about 30 minutes before serving.

3. Store tightly sealed in the refrigerator for up to 5 days.

TIP: For more flavor (and a little extra effort), use Kalamata olives in place of the black olives. Pit them and chop finely.

Per Serving (about 2 tablespoons): Calories: 53; Protein: 0g; Total fat: 5g; Total carbohydrates: 2g; Fiber: 1g; Sugars: 0g; Sodium: 216mg; Iron: 1mg

Easy Ponzu Sauce

Prep time: 10 minutes | Makes 4

Ponzu is a popular Japanese soy and citrus condiment. It has a bright and briny flavor that's perfect for rice, veggies, fish, or Ponzu Grilled Avocado (page 65). The typical citrus used for ponzu is yuzu, but this recipe calls for lime, which is easier to find.

¼ cup rice vinegar

1 tablespoon honey

5 tablespoons
low-sodium soy sauce
or tamari

1 teaspoon freshly
squeezed lime juice

1. In a small saucepan, heat the vinegar and honey until it simmers, stirring frequently. Let cool.

2. Whisk in the soy sauce and lime juice.

3. Store in an airtight container in the refrigerator for up to 2 weeks.

TIP: Feel free to substitute freshly squeezed lemon juice for the lime juice.

Per Serving (about 2 tablespoons): Calories: 30; Protein: 2g; Total fat: 0g; Total carbohydrates: 6g; Fiber: 0g; Sugars: 4g; Sodium: 640mg; Iron: 0mg

Cauliflower Rice

Prep time: 10 minutes | **Cook time:** 5 minutes | Makes 4

Cauliflower rice is a popular white rice substitute, especially when watching carbs. It's lower in calories than white rice, and it makes a delicious 1:1 substitute for rice in virtually any dish. Try it in Shrimp Fried Cauliflower Rice (page 91), or serve it as a tasty side dish for poultry or seafood.

2 tablespoons
   extra-virgin olive oil

1 head cauliflower, grated

½ teaspoon sea salt

1. In a large skillet, heat the olive oil over medium-high heat.

2. Add the cauliflower and salt. Cook, stirring, until tender, about 5 minutes.

3. Store in an airtight container in the refrigerator for up to 5 days or in a zip-top bag in the freezer for up to 6 months.

TIP: If a food processor is available, save time by placing the cauliflower florets in the bowl of the food processor and pulsing for 10 to 20 one-second pulses, until it is the size of rice.

Per Serving (about 1 cup): Calories: 96; Protein: 3g; Total fat: 7g; Total carbohydrates: 7g; Fiber: 3g; Sugars: 3g; Sodium: 190mg; Iron: 1mg

Orange-Cranberry Compote

Prep time: 10 minutes | **Cook time:** 12 minutes | Makes 4

Cranberries aren't just for Thanksgiving. These tart berries blend beautifully with orange and ginger, making this a super-satisfying fruit compote to be eaten by itself or mixed with plain Greek yogurt for a quick snack or breakfast. Try fresh or frozen cranberries for a tart and aromatic treat.

Juice of 1 orange

½ cup water

½ cup honey

1 tablespoon grated ginger

1 teaspoon ground cinnamon

1 (12-ounce) bag frozen or fresh cranberries

Grated zest of 1 orange

Pinch salt

1. In a large pot, bring the orange juice, water, honey, ginger, and cinnamon to a boil.

2. Add the cranberries, orange zest, and salt. Return to a boil.

3. Reduce the heat to medium and cook, stirring occasionally, until the cranberries burst, about 10 minutes.

4. If needed, mash the cranberries slightly with a spoon. Let cool.

5. Store in the refrigerator in ⅓-cup servings for up to 3 days or freeze for up to 6 months.

TIP: Add some texture by stirring in up to ¼ cup of chopped pecans just before serving.

Per Serving (about ⅓ cup): Calories: 180; Protein: 1g; Total fat: 0g; Total carbohydrates: 48g; Fiber: 4g; Sugars: 40g; Sodium: 43mg; Iron: 1mg

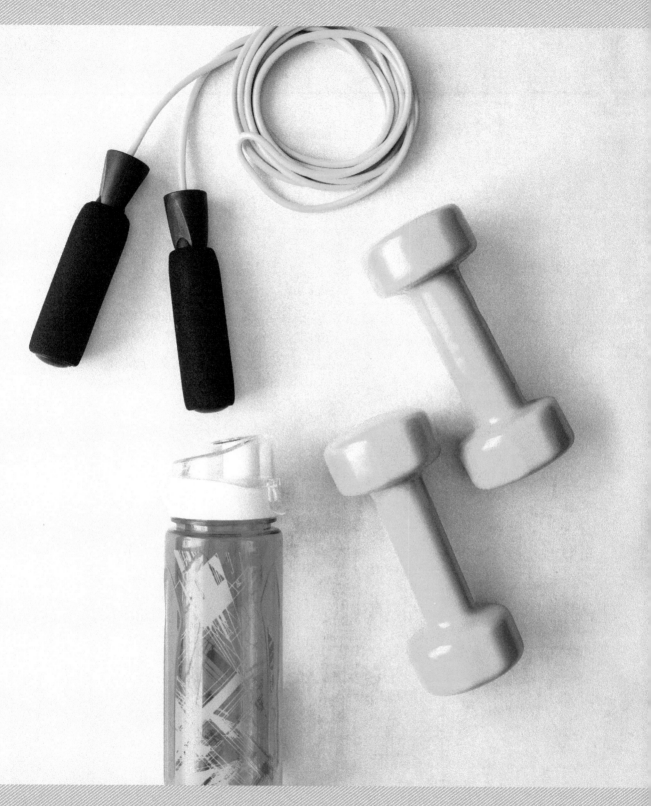

EXERCISE ROUTINES

Cardio

Walk briskly for 15 to 30 minutes. Include some light jogging if possible. Breathing should be a little harder than normal. Don't forget to stretch afterward.

Dance for 30 minutes. The style of dance should be intense enough that breathing becomes a little harder than normal. Try salsa, swing, or contra dancing. Stretching afterward is also important in this case.

Ride a stationary bicycle for 15 to 30 minutes. Try alternating between periods of higher intensity by increasing the resistance and periods of lower intensity. Riding a bike outside is another option, but make sure to increase the resistance or ride up hills to get the heart rate up. Stretching afterward is also important in this case.

Swim for 30 to 40 minutes. Try lap swimming with a couple of minutes of treading water every 10 minutes. Any style of swimming should elevate the heart rate. Stretching afterward is also important in this case.

Do step aerobics for 45 minutes. Incorporate a variety of different exercises on the step. This should cause breathing to become harder than usual. Stretching afterward is also important in this case.

Strength Training

Core Routine

Warm-up stretching

3 sets of push-ups (to failure) (page 138)

Plank (hold for 30 seconds) (page 138)

Side plank (hold for 30 seconds) (page 139)

30 bicycle crunches (3 sets of 10 reps) (page 139)

30 wood chopper exercises (3 sets of 10) (page 140)

Lower Body Routine

Warm-up stretching

30 squats (3 sets of 10 reps) (page 140)

32 lunges (2 sets of 8 on each side) (page 141)

30 wood chopper exercises (3 sets of 10) (page 140)

30 dead lifts (3 sets of 10) (page 141)

30 goblet squats (3 sets of 10) (page 142)

Upper Body Routine

Warm-up stretching

3 sets of push-ups (to failure) (page 138)

30 push press exercises (3 sets of 10) (page 142)

30 dumbbell pullovers (3 sets of 10) (page 143)

30 shoulder presses (3 sets of 10) (page 143)

Stretching

Use the following stretching routine daily or as a warm-up for strength training/cardio. This series of three types of stretches targets various muscle groups. It is ideal to hold each stretch for 15 seconds for optimal results. Breathe deeply through each stretch and be sure to monitor for any pain.

For the overhead triceps stretch, bring one arm overhead and bend it backward with the palm placed behind the head and between the shoulder blades. Bring the other arm to the elbow and gently pull the elbow behind the head.

For the seated toe touch, sit with legs extended, back straight, and feet flexed. Raise your arms above your head. Bend at the hips and reach the arms toward the toes. Hold the stretch with arms at the point where there is a stretch in the legs. It's not necessary to touch the toes.

For the standing quad stretch, while standing, reach behind and bring a foot up toward the buttocks. Grab the top of the foot and slowly pull the heel toward the buttock. Keep the knees touching. There should be a stretch in the front of the thigh. Be sure not to lean forward or to the side and to do the stretch on both sides of the body.

Stretching Routine

2 overhead tricep stretches (1 on each side, hold for 15 seconds each time)

Seated toe touch (hold for 15 seconds)

Standing quad stretch (1 on each side, hold for 15 seconds each time)

Exercises

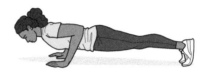

Push-Up

Start on the floor with your hands directly under your shoulders. Lift your body into a plank position with your weight evenly distributed on your hands and feet. Draw your shoulder blades back and down your back, while keeping your elbows close to your body. Lower your body until your chest touches the floor. Make sure your abs and glutes are still engaged and exhale as you push yourself up, in one straight line, to the starting position. If this is too challenging, keep your knees on the floor while performing the push-up.

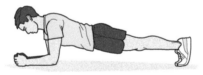

Plank

Start on your stomach on the floor. Place your forearms on the floor with your elbows aligned directly under your shoulders, forming a 90-degree angle. Raise your knees off the ground, supporting your weight on your toes and forearms. Your body should form a straight line from your head to your feet. Set your gaze at a point on the floor about a foot in front of you, and make sure your neck is in line with the rest of your body. Breathe as you hold this position, squeezing your core and glutes, for the allotted time period.

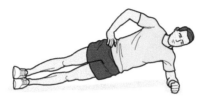

Side Plank

Another core classic and a plank variation that focuses more on the oblique muscles on either side of your central abdominals. Keep the buttocks tight, and prevent your torso from sagging to get the most out of this exercise.

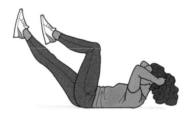

Bicycle Crunch

Start by lying on your back on the floor. Bring your knees to your chest and place your hands behind your head, interlocking your fingers. Lift your shoulders off the floor, tighten your abs, and tuck your chin into your chest. Touch the inside of your right arm to the inside of your left thigh while straightening your right leg. Alternate and touch the inside of your left arm to the inside of your right thigh while straightening your left leg. This counts as one repetition.

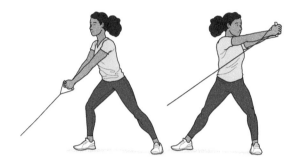

Wood Chopper

A slightly more dynamic movement that works the rotational functionality of your core and mimics chopping a log of wood. You can start with little to no weight until you feel comfortable and progress from there. Start the move with feet shoulder-width apart, back straight, and slightly crouched. If you are using weight, hold it with both hands next to the outside of either thigh, twist to the side, and lift the weight across and upward, keeping your arms straight and turning your torso such that you end up with the weight above your opposite shoulder.

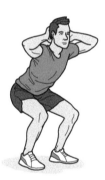

Squat

Start by standing with your feet hip-width apart or slightly wider. Extend your hands straight out in front of you for balance. Brace your abs and sit back and down like you're sitting into an imaginary chair. Keep your chest up and look straight ahead. Go as far down as you can without dropping your chest. Once you reach your depth, press through your heels and spring back into the standing position, squeezing your glutes at the top. This counts as one repetition.

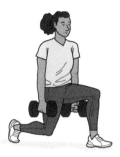

Dumbbell Walking Lunge

Start upright with a dumbbell in each hand and feet in your usual standing position. Step forward with one leg and sink down until your back knee is just above the ground. Remain upright and ensure the front knee does not bend over the toes. Push through the heel of the front foot and step forward and through with your rear foot. Start with no weights, and add weight as you feel comfortable.

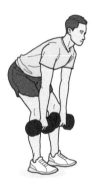

Romanian Dead Lift

Unlike the squat and lunge, the Romanian dead lift puts the primary emphasis on the rear muscles of the legs (hamstrings). Stand in a similar starting position to walking lunges, but this time you will hinge at the hips and push your buttocks and hip backward while naturally lowering the dumbbells in front of you. Squeeze your buttocks on the ascent back to the starting position. You can also do this exercise on one leg to improve balance and increase core activation—however, you may need to use lighter weights.

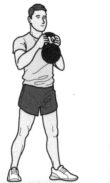
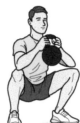

Goblet Squat

Start your stance with feet slightly wider than shoulder width and a dumbbell held tightly with both hands in front of your chest. Sit back into a squat, hinging at both the knee and the hip joint, and lower your legs until they are parallel to the ground. Push up through your heels to the starting position and repeat. Use a chair to squat onto if you don't feel comfortable.

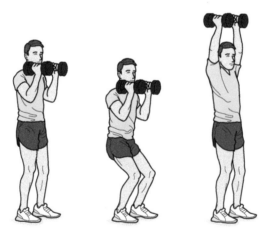

Push Press

This is essentially a combination move incorporating a partial squat and a dumbbell shoulder press. Using a weight that you are comfortable with, stand feet slightly beyond shoulder width, with light dumbbells held in a pressing position. Descend for a squat to a depth you feel comfortable with, and on the ascent simultaneously push the dumbbells overhead.

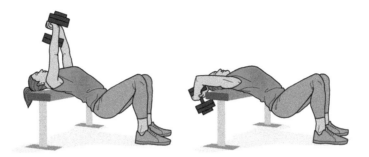

Dumbbell Pullover

Stand up a dumbbell vertically on a flat bench. Lie perpendicular to the bench and keep only your shoulders and upper back on the surface. (Your head should be off the bench.) Your hips should be below the bench and your legs bent. Plant your feet firmly on the floor. Hold the dumbbell with your palms pressing the underside. Slightly bending your arms, raise it above your chest. This is your starting position. While keeping your bent arms locked in the starting position, slowly lower the weight in an arc behind your head until you feel a good stretch across your chest.

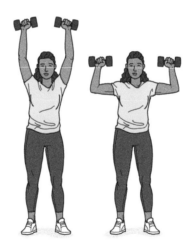

Shoulder Press

Start by standing with your feet hip-width apart and a dumbbell (or other sturdy weight) in each hand. Raise the weights to shoulder height and bring your elbows to a 90-degree angle. Brace your abs and extend through your elbows to raise the weights together directly above your head. Pause at the top and then slowly return to the starting position.

RESOURCES

Food and Drug Administration: "7 Tips for Cleaning Fruits, Vegetables"
fda.gov/consumers/consumer-updates/7-tips-cleaning-fruits-vegetables

JHEP Reports: "Non-alcoholic Fatty Liver Disease: A Patient Guideline"
doi.org/10.1016/j.jhepr.2021.100322

Mayo Clinic: "Nonalcoholic Fatty Liver Disease"
mayoclinic.org/diseases-conditions/nonalcoholic-fatty-liver-disease
/symptoms-causes/syc-20354567

National Institute of Diabetes and Digestive and Kidney Diseases: "Definition & Facts of NAFLD & Nash"
niddk.nih.gov/health-information/liver-disease/nafld-nash/definition-facts

National Institutes of Health: "Fighting Fatty Liver: Steps against a Silent Disease"
newsinhealth.nih.gov/2021/10/fighting-fatty-liver

U.S. Department of Veterans Affairs: "Non-Alcoholic Fatty Liver Disease: A Patient's Guide"
hepatitis.va.gov/pdf/non-alcoholic-patient-guide.pdf

REFERENCES

American Academy of Orthopedic Surgeons. "Safe Exercise." Accessed February 7, 2021.
orthoinfo.aaos.org/en/staying-healthy/safe-exercise.

MEASUREMENT CONVERSIONS

VOLUME EQUIVALENTS	U.S. STANDARD	U.S. STANDARD (OUNCES)	METRIC (APPROXIMATE)
LIQUID	2 tablespoons	1 fl. oz.	30 mL
	¼ cup	2 fl. oz.	60 mL
	½ cup	4 fl. oz.	120 mL
	1 cup	8 fl. oz.	240 mL
	1½ cups	12 fl. oz.	355 mL
	2 cups or 1 pint	16 fl. oz.	475 mL
	4 cups or 1 quart	32 fl. oz.	1 L
	1 gallon	128 fl. oz.	4 L
DRY	⅛ teaspoon	—	0.5 mL
	¼ teaspoon	—	1 mL
	½ teaspoon	—	2 mL
	¾ teaspoon	—	4 mL
	1 teaspoon	—	5 mL
	1 tablespoon	—	15 mL
	¼ cup	—	59 mL
	⅓ cup	—	79 mL
	½ cup	—	118 mL
	⅔ cup	—	156 mL
	¾ cup	—	177 mL
	1 cup	—	235 mL
	2 cups or 1 pint	—	475 mL
	3 cups	—	700 mL
	4 cups or 1 quart	—	1 L
	½ gallon	—	2 L
	1 gallon	—	4 L

OVEN TEMPERATURES

FAHRENHEIT	CELSIUS (APPROXIMATE)
250°F	120°C
300°F	150°C
325°F	165°C
350°F	180°C
375°F	190°C
400°F	200°C
425°F	220°C
450°F	230°C

WEIGHT EQUIVALENTS

U.S. STANDARD	METRIC (APPROXIMATE)
½ ounce	15 g
1 ounce	30 g
2 ounces	60 g
4 ounces	115 g
8 ounces	225 g
12 ounces	340 g
16 ounces or 1 pound	455 g

INDEX

ABOUT THE AUTHOR

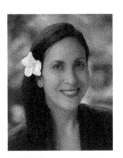

Jinan Banna, PhD, RD, is a registered dietitian and associate professor of nutrition at the University of Hawaii. She completed her undergraduate studies at the University of California, Santa Barbara, in psychology and her graduate work at the University of California, Davis, in nutrition. She conducts research on obesity prevention and teaches courses, such as introductory nutrition and community nutrition. She also helps working women lose weight so that they can feel confident and energetic and enjoy food without dieting. She offers free information on weight loss and plant-based eating on her blog, JinanBanna.com, as well as individual and group nutrition coaching. Her approach to weight loss takes enjoyment of food into consideration, and she provides individualized advice for different lifestyles that focuses on sustainable changes. Coaching sessions leave women to free themselves of dieting and to feel confident eating food they enjoy and maintaining a healthy weight.

9 781638 780540